BROKEN WINGS

The Journey from Tragedy to Triumph through My Son's Traumatic Brain Injury

Twylia G. Reid

The Author's Pen

BROKEN WINGS

Verses marked KJV are taken from the King James Version of The Bible.

Published by THE AUTHOR'S PEN, LLC
Post Office Box 720798
Houston, Texas 77272
www.tapwriting.com

Library of Congress Cataloging-in-Publication Data
Reid, Twylia, 1967-
Broken Wings / Twylia Reid

Broken Wings/ 1st Print Edition *Twylia G. Reid*

ISBN: 978-0-9906711-2-1

Printed in the United States of America

FIRST PAPERBACK EDITION

Dedication

I dedicate *Broken Wings* first to My Lord and Savior Jesus Christ for giving me the courage to share this story.

Then, to my son, Mylon RaShaun Flournoy, who has shown me the meaning of true strength. First, I want to say that I am blessed to call you my son, and I am thankful that God trusted me to give you to me to love, nurture, and to cherish until He calls you home to be with Him. You may never understand just how important you are to me and how much you have taught me and shown me that FAITH is the driving force behind all successes in life.

I have watched you develop into a handsome young man whose smile brings joy to all who come in contact with you. I have watched you cry, held your hand, and given encouraging words each time I saw the need. We have traveled many miles across the world and have experienced life as mom and son on a level many may not understand. You see, I know that God knew we both would need each other in order to see His miraculous wonders come to pass in each other's life. And, through our struggles and testimonies others would be blessed.

I pray that your life be full of joy and that you will one day discover what God has destined you to do. I know then you will find unspeakable joy, and that contagious smile of yours will continue to bless millions. You are indeed destined for greatness, so keep striving and don't ever give up as you continue to soar with *Broken Wings*. Momma loves you and I will forever be your biggest fan!

Last, but certainly not least, to anyone affected directly or indirectly by brain injury, traumatic or acquired, I dedicate this book to you, as a gift of inspiration, encouragement, and motivation to know that defeat is never an option. And, prayer is indeed a powerful weapon!

ACKNOWLEDGEMENTS

There is no way I could have the strength and confidence to write this without the love, encouragement, and support of my husband, Dexter Reid, my children, NaSharee Flournoy Davenport and Mylon Flournoy, and my parents, Arthur and Vera Flournoy. God knew just who to loan me too to watch over me until He calls me home to be with him. Mom and Dad, I love you both and truly appreciate all the love and support you two have always given me. God bless you both. Nasharee, I know you had to take a back seat to Mylon after our accident. I know there were many times when I just couldn't be there when you needed me. I want to let you know that I love you very much, and I am truly proud of you and honor the woman you are today. The hurt and pain you've experienced due to many of the decisions I had to make have made you stronger. I have watched you grow and become an outstanding wife, mom, daughter, sister, and helper to many. We have laughed together, cried together, argued and made up numerous times, but always come back with I love you's. Tierra, Leah, and Dezmond are blessed to call you mom. I want to also tell my brother, Kevin Flournoy, who gave Mylon the nickname of Bolo…and my sister, EwuVonka Flournoy, thanks for allowing Mylon to be able to say that he has the best aunt and uncle ever. I know we don't see each other as often as we'd like to, but I love you both dearly. I am grateful for your patience and for always being able to make me laugh in the midst of crying as I wrote *Broken Wings*.

I want to thank Shatrece Buchanan for pushing me and for picking up the phone on January 18, 2016 and simply texting me "Have you started writing yet"? That was the beginning of the push to get up and do what I knew I had been called to do years ago, but had allowed my heartaches, loneliness, sleepless night, and low self-esteem cause me to doubt that I'd ever be able to complete such a task. Thank you for believing in me Shatrece…even when I often times didn't believe in me. I want to thank my editors, Jaleesa Sargent and Miriam Nowon, for their wisdom and expertise. Without you two on my team, I know this would have just been thoughts in my head that were screaming to come out. Your attention to detail is impeccable. I am thankful for our newly found friendship. I want to thank Mac Whitfield for his God given gift of being a seer in the spirit. The day you text me your vision for the book cover, I knew God had opened up your eyes to allow you to see into my heart and see the vision that HE had given me for *Broken*

Wings. The mantel has shifted and it's time to move forward with what God has given you now.

Thank you, Lindsy Bivens, of The Author's Pen Publishing. Your patience, prayers and heart penetrating encouragement that you probably never even knew that you were giving to me each time we talked allowed me to absorb parts of your spirit, which truly carried me many days. Your brilliant mind and compassionate heart went hand in hand with the gifts of your time, unyielding counsel, and genuine dedication to this assignment. Working with you has been an extraordinary, professional, and empowering experience that I will never forget. Thank you for bringing *Broken Wings* to print. Our divine connection on this assignment is just the beginning. I pray that God will continue to watch over you, provide for you, and bless you immensely.

A wholehearted thank you to all the doctors, nurses, therapists, pastors, mentors, friends, and military children I adopted along the way who with the strength and grace of God continues to help protect and save Mylon's life and catapult him into his destiny. Thank you to our extended families and communities for their daily support, fervent prayers, and sincere concern during this journey we call life.

P.S…Sending a huge kiss and I love you to my husband, Dexter, whose tolerance, love, understanding, and most of all sense of humor sustains me throughout this walk. Thank you for putting up with the many, many high's and low's that you inherited when you said I do. Through the many days of emotional, mental, and physical separation we encounter I want you to know that your silent frustrations…never go unnoticed. Although you were not there with us at the beginning of this nightmare, you resurfaced during a time in my life when I was broken almost beyond repair. All I can say is God truly knew. I know I don't say thank you enough, but I really do thank you for what you do. I genuinely thank God for allowing us to go through this journey from tragedy to triumph together. I wouldn't have it any other way.

I "twill" forever love you…. always! ☺

Foreword

Caring for my family has taken me down some attention-grabbing paths in life through the years. I truly love my children. Having raised them while serving in the United States Army, allowed us to travel to many places and experience many different things, some good...some not so good. But, in the end it taught us how important it is for us to love unconditionally. This journey with my son who has a traumatic brain injury has challenged, encouraged, and motivated me in ways I have never known.

Hello and thank you for reading this book. I take it that someone in your realm of life either has a brain injury, or is a caregiver of someone with a brain injury. After years of research and searching for resources to assist me on this journey to help others, I decided to write this book. *Broken Wings* is the result of daily struggles of walking through, living for, eating and breathing life with a traumatic brain injury with my now adult son. Brain injuries can happen at any time to anyone and, many times without a moment's notice. This is our story.

My name is Twylia Flournoy Reid. My husband and I live in Savannah, Georgia. We are a blended family and have four adult children, and five grandchildren. I served 20 years in the US military and retired in 2015. Mylon and I were involved in a horrific car accident in 2001 in Fayetteville, NC and he suffered a severe traumatic brain injury. For Mylon, life has been a very challenging and a demanding journey. So many things in his life were forgotten, or became so fuzzy that his recollections of events are almost unrecognizable. Often struggling to find the right word to say, worrying about if he's going to have a seizure in public, wanting to attend colleges out of state, or simply wanting so badly to be on his own and live independently are just the tip of the iceberg of things he obsesses over on a daily basis. We literally have a conversation each and every day of what college he is going to attend and how he has contacted the school to tell them that he will be attending there during their next session. Most days are a silent struggle to move forward in ways that only a select few can ever understand. I am his primary caregiver and manage his medical care, finances, his day to day going and comings, and his facilitation through brain injury back to whatever level of independence we pray that he may one day gain. He was 11 years old at the time of his accident and is now 28 years old.

Sharing with you this very personal journey that I travel as one who is a caregiver to someone with a severe traumatic brain injury has not been an easy assignment. Many days and nights of shedding tears and crying out to God have given me a strength that I never knew I possessed. Having to deal with the frustrations of not being able to find sufficient resources or having to hear no that our medical insurance does not cover some of the cognitive rehabilitation that he so desperately needs are only some of the motivating factors which contribute to my whys of writing *Broken*

Wings. Hoping to reach just one caregiver and being able to give them the will to keep striving and advocating for their love one is all I ever want to accomplish. God bless you all.

TABLE OF CONTENTS

Introduction

The Journey from Tragedy to Triumph through My Son's Traumatic Brain Injury

Who would have ever thought June 18, 2001 would be a day our lives would be changed forever? My name is Twylia Flournoy Reid, and this is the story about my son, Mylon RaShaun Flournoy, who is a severe traumatic brain injury survivor.

Mylon was an 11-year-old honor roll student who made all A's and B's in school. During this time, he was preparing to attend pre-college classes for math and science at one of the local universities. Three days out of the week, he went to the local recreation center after school where he was a part of the local basketball team. Basketball was his favorite sport in the entire world to play. He often would tell me his dream was to go to college and play. From there, he planned on being drafted into the pros. He had big plans for the future and always told me he was going to make sure I was taken care of. I walked into the rec center and he yelled out to me, "Mom, five more minutes," as he made a three pointer.

He climbed into the back seat of the car, buckled up, and began to talk about how his practice went. We were two blocks from our house when all of a sudden, a car pulled out in front of us and "WHAM!" I screamed, and that was all I remember until we came to a halt.

When the car came to a stop, glass was everywhere. I was bleeding profusely from my head, and I suddenly realized what had just happened. We had been in an accident! After looking around me, I saw people everywhere. I couldn't move at first, but slowly began to look into the back seat. What I saw was a sight that will plague my memory forever.

There in the back seat was Mylon, slumped over and unresponsive on the opposite side from where he was before the accident. I tried to kick the door open but couldn't. So I jumped over into the back seat and put him in my arms. At that time, I realized his scalp was literally hanging from his head and his skull was cracked open on the top. I placed his dangling scalp back on top of his head and could feel the fractured skull. I began to scream and pray to God for Him not to take my son away from me. As I sat in the back seat with him cradled in my arms, a gentleman opened the door and said to me, "I am a doctor, and I am here to help." I knew then God had heard me and was going to answer my prayer. He pulled me out of the car and began to work on Mylon instantly. I immediately began hearing sirens and knew the ambulances were there. There was a lady assisting me who was also crying. I didn't know what to think or do.

CHAPTER 1

Star Student

Mylon was always a brilliant kid. He always made the honor roll and was proud of his accomplishments. Even when he was in kindergarten in Columbus, Mississippi, he was a bright child who definitely wasn't shy when it came to his class work.

As he progressed through his early years in school, he received several certificates of recognition for outstanding achievements in the advanced school programs he participated in. He received academic achievement awards for the Math Club, Science Club, and even a mock medical school. Mylon loved school and was excited about each eventful day. Teachers loved his spirit and the fact that he constantly had a smile on his face. No matter what, Mylon did whatever he could to ensure his days were cheerful and full of joy. As he walked through elementary with ease, it was no secret middle school was going to be a piece a cake.

During Mylon's sixth grade year, he applied to Fayetteville State University for their summer math and science program. Once accepted into the program, he was ecstatic for the opportunity to be on their college campus during the summer. I was super excited for him because it was something he wanted to do since the program was introduced to his school the previous year. Mylon wasn't the typical middle school kid. At the tender age of 11, he was focused on his goals and the fact he was going to college as a sixth grader. Unfortunately, that didn't happen. The program was due to start on June 25th, and our accident occurred on June 18th - just seven days earlier.

CHAPTER 2

Doomsday

We walked out the recreation center together and got into our car. My now ex-husband was driving, and I was in the passenger seat. Mylon got into the back seat and buckled up as we backed out the parking spot. Traffic was steady as people were getting off work and heading home to their families. We were about seven minutes away from our house when I saw a brown Buick approaching us.

It all happened so fast, it was literally like a flash second. We turned into oncoming traffic in an attempt to avoid him hitting us, and I could see the two lanes of cars headed straight for me. Due to the Buick hitting us with so much force, it swung my car around and Mylon was knocked out of the seat belt. Mylon was now in the path of the oncoming cars! In the blink of an eye, my car literally hit the ground. It was at that moment I realized we had been in a real-life car crash. Blood, oh there was so much blood everywhere! Glass was shattered everywhere. I was afraid to look in the back seat as to what I might see. As I turned around to look, there my son sat slumped over like a rag doll. I began to cry uncontrollably as I tried to open my door to get in the back seat. I tried and tried and tried to open the door. I kicked it and beat on it with my fist, but the door simply would not budge. I immediately jumped over the seat and placed his limp, lifeless body in my arms. I noticed his scalp was literally detached from his skull. As I placed it back on top of his head, I could feel that his skull was cracked. I screamed for someone to call for help. At that moment, it all seemed unreal. My son was lifeless in my arms, covered in blood, unresponsive, not breathing, dead - or so I thought.

It felt like there were a million bystanders watching. I remember looking out the window of the back seat as I held my son's limp body, screaming for someone to call 911. I then began screaming to God and asking Him not to take my son away from me. I pleaded with Him with every inch of strength I had left in me to please bring him back and let him live. Those few minutes, which seemed like an eternity, were minutes I will never forget. I often find myself thinking back to that moment and how the pain pierced my soul that day. It was pain like I had never experienced before in my life. That conversation with God will be one I will never forget. As I held my baby boy in my arms, I cried out to God one last time and asked Him to please not to take my son from me. As I opened my eyes, there stood a gentleman leaning into the back seat. "I am a doctor, and I am here to help," he said. Next, an older woman showed up and assisted me. Blood was streaming down my face. She took off my uniform top, wrapped it around my head and began to escort me away from my car gently. I stopped and told her I could not leave my son. She reassured me and said, "They are working on him. Come with me." By this time, I could hear screeching sirens everywhere. I could hear what sounded like helicopters and even more sirens. As the older woman helped me, she wiped the blood from my face and tried her best to console me. With tears streaming down my face nonstop, all I could think about was Mylon and the image of him in the back seat of my car in my arms. I kept telling her I needed to go back and see about my son. Each time, she would gently state they were working on him. She began to give me details of what she could see going on. For some reason, I did not have the same visual as she did. To this day, I don't understand why. She began to tell me the emergency personnel were cutting my son out of the car and placing him in the ambulance. As she gave me this play-by-play account of what was going on, all I could see was my baby in my arms limp and lifeless. The sirens were piercing and becoming louder. My son was all I could think about and I had to get to him. Where was he? Why was I not in the ambulance with him? Was he dead or did they revive him? Those were the many thoughts that raced in my mind. The third emergency vehicle arrived to take me to the hospital as well. The medical personnel leaned over me and began to remove my top the older lady had wrapped around my head to stop the bleeding. As I looked to my right, there was the guy who initially caused the accident. He was sitting in his car talking with someone. I remember looking at his feet on the ground as he was sitting in the passenger seat of this car. He appeared not to have a scratch on him. I stated to the emergency personnel, "That's the guy who hit us." While they were pushing my stretcher into the ambulance, they began drilling me with questions. I never knew what happened to the older lady who helped me so diligently and kept me calm during the chaos. Nor, did I ever see the doctor who miraculously appeared on the scene to immediately begin working on my son. To this day, I do not know who either of them are, but I am forever thankful for the two of them. I truly believe in my heart they were angels sent from God.

The ambulance ride seemed like a ride of a lifetime. All I could do was think about my son and repeatedly ask if he was ok. They cut my pants off, removed my boots and quickly gave me an IV. Once again, I began to notice how much blood was covering my top. Quickly, I reverted back to questioning them about my son.

After arriving to Cape Fear Medical Center, the local hospital in Fayetteville, North Carolina, I was rolled into the ER and placed in a room. My head was pounding, but all I could do was ask if I could see my son. They rolled me into a room, and I could see so many people rushing around in a tizzy. I was dizzy and disoriented, but all I wanted to do was see my son.

At that moment, Dr. Carol Wadon, the hospital's neurosurgeon, came over and began talking to me. I could hear her speaking, but all I wanted to hear was that my son was alive and ok. Instead, she began to cry and said, "We need to operate immediately, and I need you to sign the consent forms." Before signing the consent forms, she required me to repeat everything she said regarding Mylon's condition. I could not for the life of me repeat anything she said because I lost it after hearing, "We need to operate immediately." She made another attempt to have me repeat what she stated. I remember yelling and telling her to please just go operate if they needed to. Someone helped me articulate Mylon's condition, and I signed the forms. Upon signing, Dr. Wadon quickly ran down the hall. I can still see her white coat tail as she turned away from me.

During the wait, which seemed like five lifetimes, it was discovered I acquired four broken ribs. On top of that, glass was embedded underneath my scalp due to my head hitting the windshield. Since my adrenaline was pumping on overload since I arrived, the nurses weren't surprised I didn't feel pain from the glass in my head.

I remember asking one of the nurses if I could use her phone to call my family. She insisted on calling for me, so I gave her my sister's cell phone number. She called my sister and told her we had been in a horrible accident. While talking to my sister, she walked away from me and continued her conversation. I later learned from my sister the nurse informed her about our accident and said it wasn't looking good for my son. When she walked backed into my room, she handed me the phone. I began talking to my sister, but all I could do was scream Mylon's name. I cried and begged her to come to North Carolina to be with me right there and then. She called our mom on the phone at some point. When I heard my mother's voice asking what happened, all I could do was yell out was Mylon's name. The nurse had to take her phone back and continue talking to my family on my behalf. I remember thanking her and hugging her as tears rolled down both of our cheeks. As I laid on the bed, all I could think about was whether my son was dead or alive. The image of us in the back seat while I held him in my arms was still haunting me.

Flashback scenes of what occurred started to replay in my mind. I saw the young man pulling out of his subdivision and not stopping at the stop sign like he was supposed to.

The cars heading towards us were initially heading towards me, but my baby got hit instead. I saw the glass and blood that was everywhere after the accident occurred. There were so many spectators. Some people were crying, running, or on their cell phones, while others did nothing but watch. I saw myself praying to God as I held him in my arms. Then, I started remembering how I could not open the passenger door and how I had to jump over the seat to get to Mylon.

All of a sudden, I remembered the voice of a man I heard say to me, "I am a doctor, and I am here to help." My recollection stopped there and did not go any further. Who was this man, where was he, and where did he come from? I needed to thank him for what he did. His voice was soothing. As I began to ask the hospital personnel about this man, no one seemed to know who he was or where he came from. I think of this gentleman often and wish I could just hug him and personally thank him for what he did to help my son.

As I lay there thinking about all this, the curtain to my room opened and there stood Dr. Wadon. Her eyes were bloodshot red, as if she was crying just as hard as I was. I began to scream and say, “No, no, no. Please don’t tell me my son is dead.” She walked over to me, held my hand, and gently said, “No, he made it through the surgery, but he’s not out of the woods yet.” At that moment, she and I both cried. I couldn’t help but to thank her for all she had done. She informed me he was in the pediatric intensive care recovery area, and I could see him soon.

The next step was telling my daughter, Nasharee what happened. How would I tell her about what just occurred? She worked that day, but all I could think about was what if she was in the car with us. All of a sudden, a sick feeling came in the pit of my stomach that was so unexplainable; it literally made me feel like throwing up. The same nurse who called my sister called my daughter's manager to notify him about our accident.

“Thank you for calling Foot Action, this is Nasharee. May I help you?” As I requested, the nurse asked for Nasharee's manager. Although the manager told my daughter to take the message because he was busy, the nurse was persistent and insisted on talking to him. After the manager got on the phone, she proceeded to tell him why she was calling. Upon hanging up the phone, the manager informed Nasharee that a nurse from Cape Fear Hospital called regarding our accident. By the time they finished talking, my two coworkers were there to pick my daughter up and bring her to the hospital.

She arrived in the ER filled with questions and crying uncontrollably. We attempted to calm her down several times. Once we did, she then noticed she saw me but not Mylon. She then began to ask over and over and over again where Mylon was. At this time, there were several nurses who started explaining to her that Mylon was really hurt because of the severity of our accident. She looked at me and asked once again where was Mylon. All I could tell her was that Mylon acquired serious injuries from the accident.

The time came for us to see Mylon. The hospital personnel released us from the emergency room and escorted us to the pediatric intensive care unit. Before we went in, I remember the nurse telling us to try our best not to cry because he wasn't going to look the same to us. Even though he was unconscious, they did not know for sure if he could hear us or not. While I slowly walked into the ICU room, I saw an image that would forever be imprinted in my mind, heart, and soul.

I saw my baby lying there with IV tubes in every vein in his body. He was on a ventilator and not breathing on his own. His head was covered with bloody bandages that were so thick, you couldn't even tell how many layers were there. His face was swollen; it was the size of a basketball. There were staples in a scar located in the corner of his eye; it disappeared underneath the bandages. I stood there in shock, speechless, and with tears running down my face. All I wanted to do was hold my baby boy, but I couldn't. If he actually heard my voice, he would be incapable of withstanding the stimulation to his brain.

I looked at my son as if I was looking at a stranger; so numb, helpless, clueless, and near faint. He did not look like my Mylon. No movement whatsoever. He looked lifeless and helpless. He was covered in sheets of ice. At that moment, I couldn't bear to see him in that state and I broke down. They took me out and then it was time for my daughter to go in and see him. As they walked her towards the ICU unit, she did not even make it all the way in. When she laid eyes on her baby brother lying there barely hanging onto life, she too broke down and had to be escorted out.

Later, I talked to my family and it was comforting to know they would be on their way to Fayetteville, North Carolina the next day. My coworkers took us home so we could shower and change clothes. I was still in the hospital scrubs they put me in after having to remove my bloodstained clothes. After a hot shower and changing, we went back to the hospital to finish a journey that had yet begun.

The next day, my family arrived, and boy was I glad to see them. With four broken ribs, burns on my face from the airbags, and glass imbedded in my scalp, I embraced my worried mother. Her arms around me gave me a feeling of comfort that I will never forget. My sister, brother, and father were also there with tears in their eyes, I embraced them and didn't want to let go. Them being there somehow made me believe that everything would be ok.

CHAPTER 3

That's Not My Son

The next time I saw Mylon in the pediatric intensive care unit was with my family. "Oh no," I screamed as I saw him. He did not look like my son. His head seemed to have even more bandages wrapped around it than the night before. His face was twice its normal size and almost every vein in his body had an IV bag with some type of fluid going into it. He was still on ventilator and still not breathing on his own. It was very difficult looking at him that way. He did not look like my cheerful, happy-go-lucky son I had just picked up from the recreation center a day ago. His body shivered because of the ice packs they were using to stabilize his body temperature. Every time I saw movement, I would get excited because to me he was responsive. Each time, I was let down after the nurse explained to me it was just his body's natural reaction…even in the coma. Day by day, I would stand next to his bed looking at him and hoping he would just open his eyes. I was instructed not to touch him, as he could not be stimulated in any way. It was hard watching the other mom's cradling their babies when all I could do was stare at mine.

His face was so swollen, it looked as if it could pop at any minute. I remember trying to count the number of needles I saw in his body. Those ice sheets really creeped me out because, as I stated, each time he would shiver, I'd get excited. I remember thinking to myself, "If I could just touch him." Can you only imagine?

The bandages wrapped around his head seemed to be bloodstained every time I was allowed to go in and sit with him. I knew the nurses were changing them, so it alerted me each time I'd go in and see them covered in blood. I remember always wondering why was there always so much blood. The tube down his throat looked painful, and my stomach would get filled with butterflies as I studied how the ventilator was assisting his breathing. Watching his chest rise and fall was similar to my faith at that time. Tears would run down my face as I watched my baby just lie there helpless. "Oh God," I'd cry to myself. "Please just fix this and make it all better." I'd always promise God if He'd just let Mylon live that I would do whatever it was He asked me to do. But nothing ever changed. God knew I was talking out of emotions. He knew that even though He had my attention, the words out of my mouth were still just words. You see, God was already working it out. I just couldn't see it at that moment, but oh when I did…it was a revelation that changed my life forever!

CHAPTER 4

Stat! A Mother's Prayer of Desperation

Each day, we all piled into the Pediatric Intensive Care Unit (PICU) waiting room where we slept and ate.

This is where we literally lived for the next few days. We were making chairs into beds or finding a spot on the floor. The visiting hours for the PICU were every two hours, so we would rotate in and see Mylon during each visit. We couldn't do anything more than hope and pray for any sign of progress. We kept this routine up for five days.

On the fifth day after our morning visit, we went downstairs to get food for lunch. Then all of a sudden, we heard the words, "STAT in the PICU. STAT in the PICU." I stopped in my tracks and looked at my mom and said, "It's Mylon!" My family told me I didn't know for sure and to calm down. Once again, I yelled, "It's Mylon!!!" Then I immediately dropped what I had in my hands and ran upstairs to the PICU. Low and behold, I was right. Mylon had taken a turn for the worst! The doctors informed me that Mylon's left frontal lobe had begun to swell; therefore they needed to perform an emergency operation. I panicked and began crying uncontrollably as they disconnected him from all the tubes. We sat in the hallway of the intensive care unit while they prepared him for surgery.

They rolled his still comatose body by us and stopped so I could give him a kiss on the cheek.

The night we went home to change, I had grabbed one of Mylon's pictures to take to the hospital with me. I would lay it on my chest each night as I slept. Before retreating to the surgery's waiting area, I reached into my overnight bag and took out his picture to take with me. My mother asked me why I wanted the picture, but all I could do was look at her with tear-filled eyes as we began to walk. Hours and hours went by as we waited to hear something. I sat in one spot the entire time while clutching his picture close to my heart. That whole time, I prayed as hard as I knew how and asked God to make it all better.

Time passed and my family grew weary because we still hadn't heard anything about Mylon's condition. Finally, one of the doctors came in the waiting area and told us he made it through the surgery. "Thank you Jesus," we all cried with tears rolling down our eyes. The doctor looked at me and said, "We had to remove a portion of his brain. It had started to swell and the cells had died, so we had to go ahead and remove the portion of the left frontal lobe that was swelling." As he was telling me this, all I could think about was seeing my son and whispering to him that I loved him. I had no clue what the doctor was really telling me other than they had removed a part of his brain. To be honest, it really had not processed; all I wanted to do was see him.

There was a lady my family and I noticed this entire day who was dressed in all white. No matter where we were, we noticed she always happened to be there. We really never thought much of it, but I remember it was a presence about her I couldn't explain. Later on, you will see why she was relevant to my son's healing.

Well, back into the PICU he went again. Similar to the beginning, he was covered in ice sheets and couldn't have stimulation. The time came for my family to leave, and I had to make a decision about my daughter. I had literally been sleeping on the hallway floor of the PICU with a pillow and blanket. Although I had broken ribs and was struggling to get up and down, I did what I had to do. I vowed not to leave that hospital without my son. I sat my family down and asked my sister if Nasharee could go back with her. "Of course," my sister stated without hesitation. Furthermore, I explained to her how I wanted Nasharee to have some sense of normalcy in her life, despite what was going on. To ensure this, I requested for her to go to Alabama to live with my sister until I could bring Mylon home. She understood and with tears in both our eyes, we hugged and cried. It broke my heart to send her home, as we were already on a path of trying to heal our very own rocky relationship. Even though it was one of the toughest decisions I made, I knew it was the only option at that time.

Later that evening, she went home and packed. The next day, they all returned to the hospital to say goodbye. Boy, the pain in my heart was unexplainable. I was so unsure if I was doing the right thing. Was she going to think I abandoned her? Was she going to think I loved her less than Mylon? Was she going to resent me for sending her to Alabama? Was she going to hate me later on? Did she blame me for what happened? Most of all, how were we going to mend our already rocky relationship? Lord, please help me understand what I have done to deserve this? All this and more was racing in my mind. As I sat with trembling legs and arms, I thought I wasn't going to go on, and I was literally on the verge of a breakdown. I didn't know what to do. A few more hours passed, and it was time to say goodbye to my family. Watching them drive away gave me a feeling of emptiness that took my breath away. My daughter was leaving, and I felt like the worst mom on the planet...AGAIN. I cried and stood there until I couldn't see the car anymore. As I turned to go back into the hospital, I remember feeling like I was just going to die…and maybe that I should have. It all came back to me remembering those cars heading straight towards me. I remember saying it was supposed to be me lying in the intensive care bed, not my son. I felt hopeless and worthless. What kind of mother lets this happen to her children? What kind of mother sends her only daughter away during a time when they are supposed to be mending their relationship? The more I began to think, the more I cried. My heartbeat became faster and I began shaking.

I slowly walked back into the hospital and got on the elevator. When I got upstairs, the nurse told me they were giving me a hospital room on the same floor as my son was on. I was relieved! Now at least I could lie in a bed and not sleep on the floor struggling to move with the ribs I had broken. I was able to strap a pillow around my ribcage and be comfortable to some degree. That night was one of the worst for me ever. Even though I didn't have to sleep on the floor or in a chair, I couldn't rest. My mind was racing and kept switching from my daughter to my son. I felt so alone and just wanted to vanish.

Now mind you, I was a Soldier in the U.S. Army and actually on my way from work picking Mylon up when the accident occurred. I had not been back to work but talked to my supervisor and commander by phone. They came to see me, but I was never in any condition to visit with them due to the level of anxiety I was experiencing.

The day after my family left, I was finally stable enough to meet with them and discuss what my plans were regarding work. They were very understanding and didn't put any pressure on me whatsoever about work. I know without a doubt God had touched their hearts, and everything was going to be well.

Prior to the accident, I was preparing for an upcoming promotion board. During this particular visit, my Command Sergeant Major and immediate supervisor were trying to convince me to still attend the promotion board. Even though I understood their reasons for wanting me to attend the promotion board, I was not in any condition to do so. I understood that a promotion would mean more rank and money for me. However, I was not worried about money, bills, or anything else at the time. My only concern was my son. Since I wasn't aware of what was going to happen to Mylon, they were concerned about my finances and wanted me to attend so I could get my promotable status. They were looking out for me. Once again, God was working it out, and I could not see it yet. But, I couldn't bring myself to leave the hospital. I just couldn't leave Mylon there because I vowed not to leave that hospital without him. The only time I left the hospital was to change clothes on the first night. Being the awesome leaders they were, they remained understanding and supportive. We prayed and when they left, I thanked God for answering my prayers and touching their hearts.

The next day, which was June 25th, was long and dreary. It rained nonstop. Each visit to the PICU, I would just stand there and look at Mylon. All I could do was pray to God to let him move, allow him to open his eyes, to move or anything. One of the local ministers from one of the churches had come to visit and pray with me. He gave me a bottle of oil, which had been blessed and prayed over by the elders of his church. It was good to have him and his staff to come and pray.

Now, I still had instructions to not touch Mylon. I remember it being so hard, especially having to see the other moms being able to hug and love on their kids in the PICU. I remember one visit seeing a mom actually climbing into the bed with her son and hold him, and all I could do was stand over Mylon and look at him. Each time, I was reminded that at least he was still there for me to look at. Knowing that was good enough for me. Afterall, I didn't have much of a choice.

Following each visit, I would pray and thank God for yet another visit; prior to each visit, I would ask God to show me a sign that he was getting better. Later that evening, I noticed the woman dressed in all white relocated to the same floor as us. Remember, she was the lady who appeared the day my son had his emergency surgery. She and my mom talked and her presence was always soothing whenever I saw her. Well, I saw her periodically throughout that day but never said anything to her. The main thing that stood out to me was she was dressed in all white each time I saw her. I am not sure how long she had actually been there at the hospital, but I know her presence was relevant to me for those past two days.

The rain continued to pour down that day. I remember walking up and down the hallway of the intensive care unit that evening. It was still daylight but was starting to get dark. As I walked passed her towards my room, she handed me a piece of paper that was folded. She didn't say one word to me; all she did was give me that piece of paper and walked back into her room. Well, I took the paper and went into my room. When I opened it, there was a scripture and her name. The scripture was Hosea 6:1-3 which states, "Come, and let us return unto the Lord: for He hath torn, and He will heal us; and hath smitten and He will bind us up. After two days, will He revive us; in the third day, He will raise us up, and we shall live in his sight. Then shall we know if we follow on to know the Lord: His going forth is prepared as the morning; and He shall come unto us as the rain, as the latter and former rain unto the earth." Once I read the scripture out loud, I got my Bible, found the scripture and read it out loud again. After reading, I wrote in my Bible Cape Fear Valley Hospital 6/25/01 Prophetess Thompson.

I walked out into the hallway, and she was gone just that quick. I walked down to the room she had been in, and it was empty. I went downstairs to see if I could catch her, but she was nowhere to be found. I went back upstairs and stared out the window as it poured down raining and began to pray. As the rain poured down, so did my tears. I said to God, "I need you right now. Mylon needs you right now. I am his mother and can't do anything to help him. God at this moment, I give him to you; please heal him in the name of Jesus."

As I buried my face in my hands, tears flowed because I realized the scripture was a word from God given to me by one of His angels, Prophetess Thompson. At that moment, I felt that Mylon's healing had then truly begun. I remembered the oil the minister had given me. I took the oil out, walked to the door of the PICU, prayed and anointed the door. You could actually see the imprint of a cross on the door of the PICU from the oil. I anointed my hands before I went in to see Mylon while making sure to rub his bed, ventilator and each IV bag. I vowed to do this each time I went in to see him. This visit was different than the other visits, and the nurses were not monitoring him as they normally did during the visit. When the nurses weren't looking, I took my anointed hands and laid them on his head and feet while praying to God to heal him. I also vowed to do this each time I visited him. I knew and believed in my heart that it was the right thing to do as God was healing him.

During my visit that night, I looked at my son lying there so peacefully. I knew God was with him. Before I settled in that night, I anointed him, his bed and the door to the PICU where he actually slept. God's peace was there with me while I drifted off to sleep. For the first time since the emergency surgery, I felt in my heart that all was well.

Hosea 6:1-3 had been in my heart and on my mind the entire night. Before climbing into my bed I opened my Bible and read the scripture again. However, this time slowly, meditating on every single word. It was the first night since June 18th that I actually slept.

The next day I woke up feeling refreshed. When I went in to see Mylon, they told me he seemed to be doing better, and his temperature was stable throughout the night. I was happy to hear that news and thanked God! I called my family and told them the good news. Throughout the day, I prayed and just kept thinking about the prophetess and the scripture. Each visit consisted of the same ritual; I anointed him, his bed and the PICU door. That day was peaceful, a peace that had not been like any other since I'd been there.

During my morning visit the next day, I was welcomed in the PICU with soft, soothing music coming from Mylon's bedside! The nurse told me he seemed to be breathing on his own, and they were going to lower the strength of the ventilator. My heart leaped for joy as I immediately remembered the words of Hosea, "After two days, He will revive us." My God! My son's healing was taking place right before my very eyes. I couldn't call my family fast enough to tell them the great news. I ran in my room, fell to my knees and began to thank God. I reminisced on the words I prayed after receiving the scripture from God's angel. The part where I told God, "I give him to you," kept ringing in my head. I knew God was waiting on me to trust Him, have faith and release my son to HIM. This is what God was waiting on all along.

It was a joy to hear the music playing over his bed during each visit. Although it seemed like things had taken a turn, his lifeless body still remained there; all I could do was stare at him and pray. One morning, I stood at his bedside and observed him from head to toe. He looked so peaceful. All I could do was stare into his face and hope that he would move or something. About two hours passed of me sitting by his bedside staring at him, and then astonishingly Mylon did what I had been praying to God for. He opened his eyes, placed his left hand on my face and smiled. I screamed to the nurses to come. "He's awake," I yelled as the nurses ran over to his bedside. All I could do at that moment was cry and thank God for hearing my prayers. I literally fell to my knees right there at his bed side amid all the nurses and thanked God like never before as tears flowed down my face and theirs. The nurses took his vitals while waiting for the doctor to come in. During the entire time, Mylon and I never took our eyes off one another. I was so happy my baby finally opened his eyes. After the nurses finished their evaluation, I stood over him, looked into his eyes, smiled and told him I loved him. As he looked at me and smiled, I noticed that only one side of his face moved. Only one hand and leg moved, which could only mean one thing; he was paralyzed on his right side. Although I was sad, I was happy at the same time because my baby opened his eyes, smiled at me and knew exactly who I was. In spite of all that, I looked up to the heavens and told God thanks. All I could do was think to myself that overall, today was a GREAT day. God's word of Hosea 6:1-3 had come to pass!

The next day, the doctor came to talk to me, and his news was not so good. After careful evaluations and tests, it was determined Mylon would most likely be paralyzed on his right side and possibly never walk or talk again. I calmly looked at him and told him I appreciated his opinion, but my son would walk and talk again. I told him God assured me of that. He began to tell me that in a few days, they would be transporting him to the other side of the hospital for inpatient aggressive rehabilitation. It was going to be a long road of recovery due to the severity of Mylon's brain injury. He told me it was not going to be easy, and he could not predict how well the rehabilitation would turn out. Then he turned and walked away back into the PICU. As I stood in the hallway with tears rolling down my face, all I could think about was the scripture saying, "On the 3rd day, He will raise us up." Immediately, I began to give God praise because it was the third day!

CHAPTER 5

Lonely Days and Lonely Nights

Well the next few days, I simply enjoyed being able to go into the PICU to talk to my son and hold his hand. He still could not talk to me yet, but that smile; that smile was enough to melt anyone's heart. A week passed and he continued to show progress. Then, the day came for Mylon to be transported to the other side of the hospital for inpatient rehabilitation. As the hospital staff prepared his paperwork to be transferred, one of the surgeons who operated on Mylon came out into the hallway outside of the PICU to shake my hand. He looked at me and said, "I know we aren't supposed to say stuff like this, but I have to tell you that God is truly on your side." As I looked at him with tears running down my face, I thanked him for all he had done to take care of Mylon and wished him well. They put Mylon in a wheelchair and wheeled him to his new home, where we were expected to be for the next three months. The room was super nice. I was told by the staff that it would be good to decorate his room with some of his favorite things so that it could start helping him remember some things. Therefore, I went and got his football helmet, tons of pictures of me, his sister Sharee, my parents, my sister and brother and their families, as well as some of his friends from school. I brought all of his sports stuff and many of his trophies that he won playing basketball and football. The room was starting to look like his bedroom from our condo, with the exception of this humongous bed in the middle of the floor that zipped up from the outside. I hated looking at that bed and although I knew it was for his protection, I still hated it. The first day in the new room wasn't so bad. Maybe it was because I actually slept in that awkward bed with my son. It felt so good to be able to hug my baby boy, pray with him and say our prayers together. He and I both slept good that night, and it just seemed like nothing else mattered because I knew God was indeed with us.

The next morning, the staff came in and briefed me on all that was expected to happen over the course of the next couple of months. Mylon still could not walk, talk, or do anything for himself. His schedule would be a brutal one. Days filled with therapy, every kind that you could imagine: speech therapy, occupational therapy, physical therapy, cognitive therapy.

Mylon had a feeding tube and could only eat through this tube as he was not swallowing yet. He still could not talk, and therefore had no control over his gait. They came in and fed him through his feeding tube while I watched carefully. Afterwards, they came in to wash him and get him dressed for his first round of therapy. I sat in the chair and looked at him for a good 10 minutes. His face was still dirty, his clothes were not straight, his hands needed lotion, and he was not smiling. So I wheeled him into the bathroom and washed his face and adjusted his clothes. I put lotion on his feet, hands, and face. I gave him a hug, kiss and told him how handsome he looked; he looked up at me and smiled. I didn't want him to see himself in the mirror yet, as he had a huge indention in his head due to half of his skull missing. I didn't know how he would take seeing that, so I avoided showing him his reflection.

After sprucing him up, they came to get him to take him down the hall for his first session. I stayed behind to clean his room and make his bed. I put more of his pictures up and opened his shades in his room. Afterwards, I went down and watched him as he began his journey of long days in therapy. His first session for the day was physical therapy. They sat him in his wheelchair and would throw a ball to him. He was required to catch it with his good hand and to throw it back. This took place for about 30 minutes. They would then pull him up from his chair and sit him back down for the next 30 minutes.I paid close attention to everything they did. From there, they took him to occupational therapy. They worked with him on holding a toothbrush and washing his face. After occupational therapy, he had speech therapy. Those three sessions seemed to totally drain Mylon, and he could barely keep his eyes open. So, they closed his session out for the day and wheeled him back to his room. They placed him in his bed, zipped him in and within minutes, he was fast asleep. While watching him sleep, I replayed everything that occurred during his therapy sessions.

When he woke up, he was hungry and ready to eat. I called for the nurse to bring his food, which consisted of a bottle filled with liquid. When she came in and lifted his shirt, I noticed the feeding tube started to look infected. I pointed it out to her, and she stated to me, "Oh, it's ok." However, she reassured me she'd keep an eye on it and clean it later that day or the next day. When she left the room, I examined the feeding tube and noticed that pus was oozing from it. I called the nurse and pointed it out to her. She seemed a bit irritated but got the necessary items to clean it. I watched her closely as she cleaned it. Mylon would cringe in pain as she pressed on the area surrounding the plastic part inserted into his stomach. Later that day, it was worse. I could tell it irritated him and was apparently painful. From observing the nurse, I saw exactly how to clean it. Therefore, I cleaned the site every three hours. It was indeed infected, and I was not going to sit back and watch him in pain. From that point on, I cleaned my son's feeding tube site until it healed. The nurses did not have to clean it one single time after that initial reluctant time. This incident showed me if I wanted to ensure that my son was going to get the quality of care he desperately needed, I had to do it. I was going to have to learn how to stomach some of the tough stuff, put my big girl panties on and get involved.

Each day forward until he was discharged, I did all I could to assist in the process of his healing. Our regimen consisted of the following:

- Morning: breakfast, wash up, get dressed, pray, prepare for therapy assigned for that day.
- Afternoon: lunch, bathroom, get cleaned up, nap if time permitted, pray, prepare for therapy assigned for that afternoon.
- Evening: dinner, recreation time, bath, night clothes, listen to music, watch tv, or read, quiet time, pray, sleep.

After I was assured Mylon was asleep, I would then take a breather. I would eat, shower, read, pray and sleep in the reclining chair, as uncomfortable as it was, until the next morning. When my ribs didn't ache so bad, I'd actually crawl into his bed with him, lay next to him and watch him sleep.

I literally did this every single day until he was discharged. One time, I needed to run across the street to a local retail store to purchase personal hygiene items I needed. Mylon was quietly zipped into his bed and had fallen asleep. It was a Sunday afternoon. The sun was out and it was a beautiful day. I remember thinking later that afternoon, I would take him outside for a bit of fresh air. I went to the nurses' station and told them I was going to the store across the street since Mylon had fallen asleep. The nurse on duty acknowledged what I was telling her and assured me that she would look in on Mylon while I was gone. So, I calmly got my purse and headed towards the elevator. When I arrived downstairs, I remember the urgency of wanting to finish my shopping. The sun was out and the birds were chirping; it was such a nice day to take Mylon outside. I quickly walked across the street and got the things I needed. On my way back to the hospital, I smiled as I looked up into the heavens and thanked God for such a beautiful day. I remember the sky being so blue; it was such a clear day. Having the sun on my face felt really good, as I had not been outside for almost two weeks.

When I got back to the hospital and got on the elevator, my heart was racing for some odd reason. I was anxious to get back to my baby boy. When I arrived on the floor, I thanked the nurse for watching Mylon while I was gone. Upon arriving back in my son's room, what I saw was heart wrenching and unbelievable.

Mylon awakened and used the bathroom. He defecated in his diaper, took it off and feces were spread everywhere! I screamed for the nurse, and she ran into the room. When she saw what happened, she ran back out and came back with another nurse. Needless to say, I WAS FURIOUS!!!!!!! As they began to clean up Mylon and the mess he made, all they could do was apologize over and over for not checking in on him. Again, I was furious and literally wheeled my son into the bathroom, removed all his clothing and lifted him onto his bath chair. While fully clothed, I pushed him into the shower to clean him myself. I scrubbed and scrubbed until I knew for a fact that he was indeed squeaky clean. I could hear the nurses as they were cleaning his bed saying they thought the other had come in and checked in on him. I was just gone for 40 minutes! When I came out of the shower with Mylon, I was soaking wet but it didn't matter to me. What mattered was that he was clean and now safe. After I dried my arms and removed my wet socks, I dried him and put clean clothes on him. He loved taking long showers; I think the water on his body was an experience he enjoyed. Once I got him back in his now clean, crisp bed and zipped him back in, he quickly drifted back to sleep. I then went into the bathroom, cleaned myself up and everything else as needed. After changing, I stood in the bathroom staring in the mirror thinking to myself if I truly had what it was going to take to be able to handle this. I took a deep breath and prayed to God for strength to equip me to tackle one of the most challenging things I was about to ever have to do. I knew I was going to need it to endure what was ahead.

Afterwards, I went to the nurses' station and asked to see the head person in charge. The two nurses were terrified and both assured me that I didn't need to speak to anyone because they would be more careful. I demanded to speak to someone and when I did, I requested to be able to bathe, feed, clean, change, and anything else that my son needed. My goal was to ensure he was properly taken care of, and I'd do everything in my power to make that happen. I was granted permission; the only thing I could not do was administer his medication. I was ok with that, but you better believe I was right there each time they had to.

Although it was tiring, I vowed to do this until he would be able to go home...and I did just that.

Needless to say, we weren't able to go outside that day. However, the next day was just as beautiful as the day before. After a long day of grueling therapy, dinner and a brief nap, I put Mylon in his wheelchair and took him outside in the hospital's beautiful courtyard. While we were out there, he began to look around and smile. He still had not regained movement on his right side yet. Although it was a crooked smile, it was the most beautiful smile ever. I had taken a basketball outside with us. It was his favorite sport before the accident, and he absolutely loved it! I wheeled him over to the center of the courtyard, stood in front of him and explained that I was going to throw the ball to him. I wanted him to try his best to catch it. Well, low and behold as I got ready to throw the ball, he looked up at me and the look in my baby's eyes was a look that just melted my heart. He reached out his left hand and caught the ball! The excitement he displayed was amazing! I stood there and literally threw that basketball back and forth to him for two hours straight. Even though I was exhausted, I didn't care because he was able and willing to try; I was determined to do whatever it took to help him.

As dawn approached, the courtyard lights came on and a flock of birds flew over our heads. It looked like a swarm of birds migrating from one region to another. Mylon looked up and became so frightened. He grabbed me with his left arm and buried his head into my clothes. I hugged him tight and assured him that he was safe, and I'd never ever let anything hurt him. He held my hand and gave me that smile, as I wheeled him back inside to retire for the evening. Even through all that occurred, God was constantly reassuring me He was there with us both.

Months went by and our routines became more and more familiar. Mylon regained his strength little by little but was still not walking or talking. One morning, we got ready for his occupational therapy appointment. Mylon was fed and dressed, and we were just waiting for them to come to the room to get him.

I had the tv on in the room, and we were watching some music videos. As Mylon sat in his wheelchair, his head began to move to the music and he seemed to be really enjoying it! His left leg was moving to the music, he was smiling and appeared to be trying to dance. I walked over to him and asked him if he liked the music that was playing. He looked at me and nodded his head. I stood in front of him, held his hands and danced with him like we were actually on a real dance floor. It was amazing! Our dance session lasted for about 10 minutes until his occupational therapist arrived. I got him up to go use the bathroom, and upon standing him up, he looked at me and made an attempt to move his right leg! "OMG," I screamed. "He's trying to walk." It was a quick leg movement, but it was enough to give me hope. It was enough for me to remember what God promised me and enough to show me that my baby boy was indeed on his way to recovery! When the therapist heard my scream, he ran into the room to hear about what I just witnessed. He took Mylon down to the OT room and began his therapy for the day. It was a great day filled with hope and dreams for the future. Later that evening, I sat in front of Mylon and began to talk to him. I talked to him as if he understood every word I was saying to him. Although he was unable to answer me, in my heart, I knew he understood every word I was saying to him. I looked at him and told him that he was going to walk again. No matter what it took, I wanted him to trust God and never give up.

After dinner, I wheeled Mylon down to the large indoor gym and stood him up in front of me. I had observed someone doing this technique with him and it seemed to have positive lasting effects. I placed the huge support belt that the therapist used around us both. I secured it tightly, faced Mylon towards me and placed his feet on top of mine. We took one step backwards at a time. The first couple of attempts he almost fell, none-the-less, after the third attempt he had grasped the concept of what to do. This gave him the sensation that he was taking forward steps. My God, was he heavy! But after taking each step, I'd pray and ask God to give me the strength to take another one. It was awesome seeing him standing up. Although it was with me assisting him, just to see my baby trying his best was the greatest feeling in the world. We would do this several days a week, and it just became something we did because he really enjoyed it; despite how tiresome it was for us both.

Six weeks of therapy passed. This particular morning Mylon's therapist came to pick him up for his morning session. Although, this seemed like a normal morning what occurred that day was far from normal. I was in his room tidying up before I went down to join him. All of a sudden, not only did I see Mylon walk past the room, but I saw him running past the room! I ran to the door because I truly thought I was seeing things. Immediately after, his therapist was chasing him while yelling," Mylon, stop!" I couldn't help but to laugh hysterically. Who would've thought that my son, who was paralyzed and in a wheelchair since we arrived, would be running from his therapist! "Thank you Jesus," I wept uncontrollably with tears of joy. Once the therapist caught up with Mylon, he assisted him back to the OT room. Wow, the smile on Mylon's face was the biggest one we had seen yet. He was thrilled at what he accomplished, although not understanding how dangerous it was, he was still thrilled….and heck we all were!

Well, from that day on, no more wheelchair was needed unless it was required! There was however a special chair he still had to use in the shower as a precautionary measure, in case of an accidental fall. But it was ok; Mylon didn't mind that at all. Boy, did it feel good seeing him walk beside his therapist for each session, rather than being in a wheelchair. Again, each day it was just another reminder of God's healing power. Each night, we thanked God for healing him and expected God to do the rest.

Each night after Mylon went to bed, it was such a lonely time for me. I'd think about my daughter and how she was doing. I'd feel so bad about having to send her to live with my sister. Although I was indeed thankful for my sister being able to take her, the guilt just overwhelmed me each and every day. Sometimes, I wondered if she resented me for sending her to live with her aunt. I never want her to feel like I love her brother more than her because I love my children all the same. If she really knew how much I loved her, she'd never

ever really comprehend it. All these thoughts clouded my mind each and every night. I felt lost and burdened. Being in an abusive marriage and having the abuser leave during the middle of this was enough to drive anyone insane. Him leaving was probably a blessing in disguise. Lord knows being jumped on in the hospital, sometimes even in front of Mylon, and having to hide it from others was just too much to deal with. This toxic relationship was truly something I could not endure; especially while having to watch my baby boy go through the toughest time in his life. After all, he was fighting for his life. Actually, so was I.

Although Mylon was now walking, he was still not talking. His time with the speech therapist was always one that I looked forward to each day. I would watch her closely and imitate the tactics she used during her sessions with Mylon later on each evening.

One morning while waiting for a therapy session to begin, I sat with Mylon on the bed while holding a pad and pencil. I handed it to him, and he began to scribble on it. He scribbled quite a bit and once he finished, he looked at me and blurted out, "Momma!" I jumped off the bed, yelled for the nurse to come here and told her, "He said momma!" It was as if in his effort to try so hard to speak, he forced his mouth to say it. I can't even explain to you how I felt at that moment. The speech therapist came into his room and as I explained to her what happened, she began to explain to me what happened. Mylon's desire to speak triggered a response and forced his brain to say the word momma. Boy, I tell you I cried like a baby as I fell into her arms. Little did she know, what she had told me was that my baby boy actually knew who I was. He desired so badly to acknowledge me, his will power to speak forced his brain to actually do it.

Now, this was the breakthrough we had all been waiting on. It was wonderful. Mylon did not really comprehend what happened, but it was comforting to us. Even though we had not yet won the war, we were definitely winning this battle. After each battle won, Hosea 6:1-3 would ring out louder and louder. God was doing it just like He said...miracle after miracle after miracle.

CHAPTER 6

Starting Over...A Caregiver's Nightmare vs. A Caregiver's Dream

After months of inpatient rehabilitation, it was time for Mylon to be discharged. I attended several meetings with the hospital staff on what the next step for Mylon would be. I was still on active duty and had not been to work the entire time my son had been in the hospital. My former husband left me and returned to his hometown, and my daughter was still living with my sister. My chain of command had been amazing. You couldn't tell me God wasn't real. Witnessing God perform miracles in my son over the past several months was awesome all by itself. To have military superiors support me the way they did was unheard of. Not one time did they try and force me to leave my son's side. Not a day went by that they didn't contact me to see if I was ok or if we needed anything. Not once did they ever not show love and support. It was amazing. I knew a decision had to be made about our next step.

The hospital's rehabilitation staff and I had a meeting about two weeks before Mylon was to be discharged. During this meeting, I found out that outpatient rehabilitation would only be provided ONCE a week at Duke University.

I was simply blown away! By this time, Mylon was probably able to speak about five words. You know, simple words like momma, yes, no, give me, and things like that. I knew if he didn't receive more therapy than that, his progress would slow down; I just couldn't fathom the thought of that. Therefore, I told them to give me a week to see what I could come up with. They agreed, and to the drawing board I went. I spent countless hours of researching and trying to find a location where my son could get a more extensive outpatient rehabilitation program.

I made call after call to every place I found that offered brain injury services. I knew Children's of Alabama was a great place. I often heard of many wonderful things about them, but it was where my now ex lived and God knows I didn't want to go there. On the bright side, it was where my sister lived and I could get my daughter back. This would be the perfect opportunity for her to be reunited with her brother and I. I contacted the hospital, and they told me about an awesome outpatient program that was perfect for Mylon's needs. It was a five-day a week program, where he would come each morning and I'd come back to pick him up at the end of the day. During the day, he would receive extensive treatment and various services, which included speech, occupational therapy, and physical therapy. It was just what he needed, but there was one problem. Our insurance would not pay to transport him there. I was faced with one of the toughest decisions I ever had to make regarding my son's recovery. It was one that would forever change his life and mine.

Well, I met with the rehabilitation staff and informed them of my decision to turn down the therapy at Duke. I told them I was aware that my insurance was not willing to transport Mylon to Alabama, but I was prepared to do what needed to be done. The next week was discharge week. Each day when Mylon went to his final sessions, I packed his things in his room. All the pictures and familiar things throughout his room were neatly placed in a huge box. His football helmet, basketball jerseys, pictures of friends and family that helped in his healing process were all put away. That night, Mylon and I walked around downstairs in the courtyard. We sat and both just stared at its beauty. I imagined that he was probably thinking about the same things I was. We spent many evenings throwing the basketball out there for hours at a time. He probably saw me shed tears of joy after each tiny milestone, and those tears were shed right there in that courtyard. It was definitely a bittersweet moment. While we sat there, a swarm of birds flew over us, and I glanced over at my boy. He lifted his head up and smiled. All I could do was simply smile back and tell him how much I loved him. I grabbed his hand and we walked back inside.

We then walked into the gym where I reminisced even more. Many evenings were spent there teaching Mylon how to walk again; his feet on top of mine while taking one step at a time. Tears began to roll down my face as I thanked God for just being who He was and all that He had done for us both.

We went upstairs to prepare for our last night staying at Cape Fear Medical Center. I prayed with Mylon and zipped him in his bed. He had a very visible indentation in his skull, the size of half a cantaloupe. While admiring my baby boy, he smiled at me with tears in his eyes. God continuously showed me signs that everything would be ok

We both had a good night's sleep. Mylon slept throughout the whole night, and amazingly so did I. I got up and quietly got our things together without trying to wake him. I went into the bathroom to get dressed and looked into the mirror at myself. I was not the same person I was months ago. My hair had grayed; my eyes had bags under them. Several pounds were lost, and I was now bald where the glass was embedded in my scalp. "Wow,"

I thought to myself. “I got to start combing my hair a different way to hide this.” I literally stared at myself for about 10 minutes thinking about what my next move was about to be like. I was literally preparing to drive my brain injured son to Alabama from North Carolina all by myself. We had no place there to stay yet, and I had not told my chain of command yet. What the heck was I thinking?

After I got dressed, the nurses came in with Mylon’s breakfast. They checked the site where his feeding tube was removed about three weeks prior. It looked awesome. Due to the problems he had with his gait and his inability to verbally communicate, he could only consume soft, puréed foods. He ate all his breakfast, I got him dressed and it was time to sign the papers to leave.

Mylon walked over to the nurses’ station to say goodbye. One of the nurses began to hug him, he leaned forward and tried to look down her shirt. I was so embarrassed. They already informed me about some of the behavioral changes associated with brain injuries. But, I had not actually seen him do this before! At that moment, a smidgen of doubt entered into my mind. I honestly thought to myself, am I going to be able to handle this?

After all the goodbyes and taking care of all the discharge procedures, it was time to leave. It seemed so bittersweet because this had been our home for the past four months. They put Mylon in a wheelchair and wheeled him down to the elevator. Fear gripped me like never before when we approached the elevator. Although I had been heavily involved in Mylon's daily care, it all seemed surreal. My son, who was once a quiet honor student, was now a brain injury survivor with years of recovery ahead of him. I took a deep breath and just whispered to myself, "Lord, help me please."

The elevator ride was one I'll never forget. The doctor's last words to me were, "This is probably the most your son will recover considering the severity of his injury." But then again, the voice of a surgeon who operated on him was also in my ear. He said to me, "God is truly on your side." The nurse was talking to me, but all I could do was watch her mouth move. I was numb. We got to the first floor and exited the elevator. I pulled the car up so we could load Mylon inside. We got Mylon positioned in the backseat and as I hugged the nurse, she and I both cried. I thanked her, and she wished us well. I watched the nurse waving in the rearview mirror while I drove off. Once we got to the stop sign in the parking lot, I turned back and asked Mylon was he ready to go. He nodded, gave me the biggest smile ever and we drove off.

The ride from the hospital to our condo was interesting. Mylon seemed to be excited about everything he saw: the traffic lights, the stores, the cars, and just every little detail. Paranoia struck me; I kept watching him in the rearview mirror to make sure he was seated and secure in his seat belt. I was relieved when we made it home. When we arrived at our condo, I sat in the car and just stared. I literally could not move, and tears began to roll down my face. It hit me like a ton of bricks how our lives were indeed changed forever and what was about to happen.

I helped Mylon out the car and helped him into the house. After we got in, I got him situated in my bed. He seemed exhausted! It dawned on me that our bathroom was not like the bathroom in the hospital! How was I going to bathe Mylon? Well, I was too tired to figure it out. I washed him up and put on his night clothes. Without hesitation, he went straight to sleep.

Finally, I was able to sit down for a few minutes and think about our next move. There I sat on the living room floor with my face buried in my hands. All I could do was cry and pray. I got up checked on Mylon, and he was still sound asleep.

Oh, how I longed for a nice, long bath. Plenty of showers were taken, but I never had the opportunity to take a bath while Mylon was in the hospital. Being able to soak in the hot bathtub felt like heaven to me. Afterwards, I contemplated how I was going to tell my bosses about getting Mylon to Alabama. I called my supervisor and told him I needed to speak with my entire chain of command the next morning. As usual, I had their support. Darkness fell upon me and as always, I decided to lean on God. I read my Bible and said my prayers until my soul felt at ease. Once I felt comfortable, I climbed into my bed and we both slept throughout the whole night.

I awakened refreshed. God dispatched His angels to watch over us, and I thanked Him for it. We had a long road trip ahead, and God was right on time with our good night's rest. I got up and dressed Mylon for the day. He seemed happy and content. His happiness was enough for me to feel happy and content. I walked with him into the bathroom. After using the bathroom, we walked over to the sink to brush his teeth and wash his face. He began to cry once I removed his bicycle helmet and he looked in the mirror. The hurt in his eyes pierced my heart so bad. From that point on, I would have to be his strength until he was able to be that for himself. I begged him not to cry and let him know he was handsome. My goal as a mother was to reassure him that God was going to make everything better.

Mylon ate breakfast while I packed our bags. Everything was still all unclear because I had no idea where we would stay. On top of that, I didn't know how I'd get what we needed to get into the program at the Children's Hospital. All I knew was I was going to do it with God's help.

Once we finished our breakfast and had a bathroom run, we loaded everything in the car. I situated Mylon in the backseat of my Pontiac Bonneville, while assuring my condo was secure. Then, we headed on base to talk to my chain of command. So many questions raced through my mind; what was I going to say? What if they think I am crazy or out of my mind? Nonetheless, I pushed forward. I arrived to my office, got Mylon out the car and went inside. It was great seeing everyone. Their prayers and endless acts of kindness during the hospital stay meant the world to me, and I was finally able to thank them. While walking into the office, I knew Mylon would need supervision while I spoke with our Command Sergeant Major and office supervisor. One of my coworkers happily agreed to sit with Mylon. I remember closing my eyes and saying a quick prayer before walking into the meeting.

It was just a good feeling of ease when they began to tell me how good it was to see me and my son. I expressed to them how truly grateful I was for all the love, care, and support they had shown me during the hospital stay. After all that was done, I suddenly felt a huge lump in my throat. They asked what was the next step in Mylon's progress, and here is where I had to pull up my big girl panties once again and tell them the move I had to make. I looked at them both and again thanked them for all they had done for me. I explained how the local area had limited outpatient care for my son, and the amount of care he needed was not being offered locally. After listening very attentively to what I was saying, my Command Sergeant Major looked at me and said, "Well Soldier, what are you going to do next?" I took a deep breath and pulled out an index card where I had written my full name and cell phone number on it. There was a space left for my address, however I provided an address and phone number for my parents and sister. At this point, I slowly handed it to my supervisor and told them I was leaving. To ensure they understood my logic, I explained the brain injury day treatment program at Children's Hospital in Alabama. Furthermore, I went into detail about how Tricare agreed to pay for the treatment but not the transportation. I asked for their blessings and told them I understood I was a Soldier, but I had to take care of my son. Once I got settled into a place, I promised to provide them with my contact information. With tears in my eyes, I asked for their blessings again. To my surprise, my Command Sergeant Major looked at my first line supervisor, and they both nodded. I jumped up and before I knew it, hugged them both. By this time, we were all crying. I walked out of that office feeling like I just accomplished the biggest task on Earth. I said my goodbyes and thanked everyone for their prayers and support.

When we got to the car, I looked at Mylon with his bicycle helmet on. As he was holding my hand, I looked up towards heaven and said, "Ok, God." I put Mylon in the back seat of the car, strapped him in with his pillows and blankets, and headed towards the highway. Where we would stay, how this was going to work, or what the next move was…I didn't have a clue. All I knew was I had placed all my trust in God and believed He wouldn't bring us this far to leave us.

CHAPTER 7

FEAR: False Evidence Appearing Real

Our trip from North Carolina to Alabama was typically about 7 and a half hours, but this time it turned out to be a 12 hour drive! Although I had to stop every hour so Mylon could stretch and use the bathroom, I didn't complain one bit. During the times he slept, I was able to drive a little bit more. Even then, I'd stop to wake him up so he could stretch. The drive was peaceful. I remember just being able to talk to God and listen to music as we traveled to what was then the unknown. There were times when a certain feeling would come over me. I'd start to think about how I was going to make it and how our lives had changed. My baby boy was indeed a true miracle.

Several thoughts raced through my mind about how my daughter was going to handle all of this. Her life had been shifted tremendously due to everything that occurred. I couldn't help but to think about what was now considered normal for her. In spite of all the fear and doubt, only two things kept me positive; the look on Mylon's face each time I looked into the back seat and the vision of my daughter.

We arrived at one rest stop so Mylon could use the bathroom, and he seemed so happy. He was smiling and was actually dancing, and I couldn't help but laugh. Once I got him back in the car, I asked him if he wanted to dance. He looked at me and said yes. I turned the radio up, and we both began to dance. It was one of the best feelings ever to see his arms and legs just moving. The emotions I had at that moment were indescribable, and I couldn't help but to cry. It was one that I vowed to hold on to forever.

The remainder of the ride was peaceful and full of thoughts. What was Alabama going to be like? Where were we going to live? Was the transition from inpatient care to outpatient care going to be smooth for us, especially for Mylon? Was my daughter going to be able to adjust to her "new" baby brother? Thoughts here, thoughts there, thoughts everywhere! But one thing was for certain; no matter what we had to face, we would all do it together.

When we arrived into Alabama, the sun was beginning to set. The sky was beautiful. The colors of the sky looked as if God painted a picture just for me, and it was simply breathtaking. "Heaven is speaking," I thought to myself as I took in its beauty. I thanked God for safe travels. Then I looked at Mylon and said, "Son, our journey is about to begin." The look he gave me was confirmation that he understood what I meant. As usual, he showed me that beautiful smile and nodded. That to me was the sign I needed; all would be well.

CHAPTER 8

FAITH: Forwarding All Issues To HIM

I contacted my sister to notify her that I was in Alabama and was anxious to see my daughter. At some point, I knew I had to see her, but I was extremely nervous. Often, I wondered would her brother recognize her, or if she'd cry once she saw him. What if she had questions that I couldn't answer? Living with my sister was a big adjustment for her. So many thoughts were on my mind.

We settled in for the night at a local hotel, and I prayed the next day would be a productive one. I needed to get Mylon out of that car and inside so he could relax. Once we got settled into our hotel room, Mylon sat on the bed and just looked around. By the look on his face, he didn't know where we were or why we were there. I got him ready for his shower, changed his clothes and ordered us food to eat. After he ate, I gave him his medicine and tucked him into bed. I prayed over him, and he stilled seemed perplexed about what was going on. But nonetheless, he hugged me; I kissed his forehead and told him good night. He scooted over, and I knew he wanted me to sit on his bedside until he fell asleep. He was unfamiliar of where he was or what was going on, so I was his source of comfort. With my back against the headboard, he wrapped his hands around mine and laid his head against my arm until he was sound asleep. For an entire hour I watched him as he lay there postured as a newborn baby just brought home from the hospital. At that moment, I closed my eyes and did what I had been wanting to do since all this happened. I asked God why did He let this happen to my son, and why did He let this happen to me. A lump in my throat grew larger as I wept. All I wanted to do was scream as loud as possible, but I couldn't.

Slowly, I got up to prepare for bed. Although I wanted to shower, I decided to simply wash up because I was scared. Showering meant I would have to close the bathroom door, and I didn't want to take a chance on Mylon falling out the bed. I had placed pillows around him to act as a shield until I got ready to lie in bed. The pizza I ordered was cold, and I didn't want to turn on the microwave because I thought it might wake him up. So, I ate it cold. Boy, was I exhausted. After finishing my pizza, I brushed my teeth and said my prayers. I walked over to the bed to remove Mylon's bicycle helmet and the pillows surrounding him. While sitting on the bed thinking about the next day's events my heart began racing due to the joy and excitement I felt knowing I would see my daughter! I climbed into the bed and before I knew it, I was asleep.

Morning came before I knew it. When the sun shined into the room through the blinds, I felt God communicating with me. He was reassuring me that He was there and would be with us to tackle the obstacles to come. Mylon was sleeping sound, therefore I didn't want to wake him up. He slept in until about 11:00 a.m.

While he was asleep, I called my sister to talk to her and my daughter.

The excitement in my baby girl's voice filled my heart with joy, and it brought tears to my eyes. So much guilt and pain consumed me about having to send her to live with my sister. I hated to interrupt her life that way. She never knew how much I wrestled with having to make the decision to send her to live with my sister. I felt awful. We had already been apart due to her living with her father for a little while. Many bad decisions were made on my behalf regarding the men I brought into my life. It had caused so much pain for her and Mylon. Having to send her to live with my sister was just one more thing I constantly beat myself up about. I told her what my plans were for the day and that I'd be there when she got out of school. It was so good hearing the joy in her voice. We said our I love you's, and she headed off to school for the day. I gave my sister a rundown of my agenda for the day and told her I'd be in touch with her throughout the day.

Afterwards, I got Mylon dressed, fed and out the door we went. Our first stop would be The Children's Hospital in downtown Birmingham, Alabama. This hospital was one of the best in the world. I already spoke with them about the amazing outpatient brain injury day treatment program they had. And, they seemed to have all Mylon needed for his next phase of his recovery. I was excited to get him started. We arrived at Children's Hospital, parked and I helped Mylon out the car. He looked nervous and afraid. I assured him that I'd be right there with him and that I'd never leave him.

We walked through the doors of the hospital hand in hand. There seemed to be hundreds of people moving about the huge lobby. I asked for directions to the brain injury department, and we walked there slowly. People stared and pointed when they saw Mylon walking by with his bicycle helmet on. With every step, he squeezed my hand a little tighter. I kept assuring him that I was with him and would not leave him. When we approached the brain injury department, I gave Mylon a hug and kiss. Before we proceeded, I was waiting on him to show me that smile. I told him Jesus was with us, therefore we had nothing to fear. Once he smiled, we walked into the clinic. I introduced Mylon and myself, filled out paperwork and waited for the intake nurse to call his name.

What seemed like an eternity was only actually 20 minutes. "Mylon Flournoy," the nurse called. We got up and walked to the area where she took his vitals. Afterwards, I began to explain to her why I had chosen their hospital and program. She informed me they did have room for him, and he would be ok to start in three days! I was so excited. I knew they had a wonderful recovery success rate and felt happy to know that Mylon would be getting the treatment he needed. Mylon didn't quite understand what was going on; all he knew was his mommy was excited and happy. The nurse explained to me he would have a program tailored specifically to his needs. On top of that, he would be there five days a week from 8:00 a.m. to 4:00 p.m. That would give me time to look for a place for us to stay and get situated. We walked out of the hospital, and all I could do was thank God for making a way. Without a doubt, He was indeed with us! While I hugged Mylon, I expressed to him he was going to be alright and was in the best hands now. Before going to see my baby girl, we went to eat and to take care of a few loose ends.

When I saw Sharee, we both cried and were happy to see each other. She hugged Mylon so hard, I had to remind her she needed to be careful with how she handled him. It felt so good having us all together again. Even though she was living there with my sister, it just felt so good to hold her again and see her face. I shared with them the great news about Mylon's treatment and the fact we'd be together again. Mylon was content seeing everyone together and seemed to have no care in the world. Life at that moment was great, and I felt like I was definitely going to be ok.

Night approached, and we prepared to go back to our hotel. We hugged and said our goodnight's before Mylon and I departed to the hotel. As we were riding to the hotel, I had the radio on and I noticed that he was nodding his head to the music. When I turned up the music, he began to dance like no one was watching. I laughed so hard, and it felt so good to see him so happy.

Upon arriving to the hotel, we held hands like two little kids and headed for the elevator. Once inside, the routine was repeated from the previous night. The only difference was this time when he went to sleep, there was a look of peace on his face that I hadn't seen in a while. It was one of the best feelings ever to see him this happy.

Once Mylon was asleep, the haunting thoughts of the accident once again returned. My mind raced back to June 18th and how far he had come. The images of him slumped over in the back seat of the car, the glass and blood everywhere, the angelic doctor and prophetess were just a few. God's promise to me had not been returned void. I thanked God that night and just felt a sense of peace like never before. Although I was afraid, I knew I could FAITH; Forward All Issues To Him. He was there with me! We both slept until 10:00 a.m. the next morning.

We got up refreshed and energized. I looked at Mylon and asked him if he knew what today was. He shook his head no and asked me, "What?" I told him it was apartment hunting day. He laughed at me like I had told the funniest joke he ever heard. While chuckling along with him, I grabbed the phone and scheduled viewings for four apartments.

Out the door we jotted, as we buckled up and set out on a mission. The first apartment we found was a three bedroom. I couldn't afford a three bedroom at the time, so that one was a no go. The second and third apartments were too small for the furniture I had. When we approached the fourth one, I prayed and asked God to please let this be the one. It was further than the others, but it was in a nice, quiet area. It was a two-bedroom upstairs apartment with a nice balcony; it had a huge ceiling fan and a swing. I fell in love with it and knew it was the one. The apartment manager and I completed the paperwork. Fortunately, everything went through and I walked away with the keys to our new apartment.

When we got in the car, I let out a huge sigh. It was a relief knowing that after feeling so much guilt, we would all be living under the same roof again. Mylon looked at me and smiled. That moment let me know once again that all would be well. Enthusiasm was all I felt while heading back to my sister's house to spend time with my family. Life was great, and I remember feeling like I must be really special to God.

The time with my daughter, sister, niece and nephews was great that evening. We laughed and just had an amazing time. I shared with them all the great news and all that I had planned to do. I told my daughter I wanted her to come live with us. Despite having to change schools due to our apartment being on the opposite side of town, she agreed. It felt like everything was coming together again.

The time came for Mylon and I to go back to the hotel. He had tears in his eyes and didn't want to leave his sister. It was emotional that evening, but I knew that it wouldn't be long before the three of us would be in the same place again.

When we got back to the hotel, Mylon seemed very tired and agitated. I knew it had been a long day, and this was a learning experience for us both. It was my first time realizing that long days triggered irritation and increased frustrations. Instead of letting him shower, I washed him up and put him to bed.

It was a long day for us both, so we went to bed. However, it took longer for him to fall asleep. I remember making a mental note to myself of the observation I had made earlier. I was exhausted but also happy to have been able to make such an observation. I thought to myself as I drifted off to sleep that although all my TBI training was kicking in, it was heartbreaking to see him react that way.

The next morning, I contacted my chain of command to give them my new address and phone number. I informed them about the progress I made and told them I'd be coming back there to get my things from the condo. They wished me well and told me to make sure I checked in with them periodically. As I hung up the phone, I began to cry like I've never cried before. It dawned on me how blessed I truly was and just how much God's favor was over my life. The next day would be dedicated to Mylon starting his program at the Children's Hospital. With that being said, I spent the entire morning making sure I got all he would need for his big day. In preparation for the upcoming week, I got a U-Haul for our trip back to North Carolina. We still needed to get our furniture and turn in our keys.

It was a slow, peaceful day. We didn't stay out long because I wanted to make sure Mylon had a peaceful, quiet night. We ordered food, ate and got ready for the night. Mylon and I spoke with my daughter to tell her good night. I explained to Mylon that he'd be starting his program the next day, and he wasn't too excited about it. The feeling of not completely understanding what was occurring was causing his uneasiness. As always, I assured him everything would be ok, and I'd never leave him. We said our prayers, and this time, I put on some nice soothing music to help him relax and doze off. As he slept, I wrote out all the things I needed to do while he was at his program. Time would be critical and every moment would count. I had to make sure I used that time wisely to do as much as I could. Midnight approached, and my eyes grew heavier and heavier. I quietly laid down and looked up at the ceiling. There were plenty of reasons for me to smile, and I certainly kept that smile until I went to sleep.

The next morning, I knew I had to activate my FAITH once again; Forward All Issues To HIM. Today was a big day; it marked a new chapter in Mylon's road to recovery. My focus was getting dressed and getting everything else together before waking Mylon up. Initially, he was hesitant when I woke him up, but that attitude turned around when I poured out positive energy.

Well, it was time to go to the hospital for the first day of his day treatment program. The ride was kind of quiet, and he didn't say too much. When we arrived, he held my hand extra tight as we walked into the hospital. We got inside and there were several other children there. The intake nurse greeted us with a smile. We both followed her into the back. There were tons of stations set up, several children maneuvering about, and many adult workers as well. She sat us down and went over his schedule for the day. It consisted of physical therapy, occupational therapy, speech, disability insight training, social settings training, lunch, breaks, and a list of other things. She assured me that all would be well, and Mylon would be just fine. We had a few moments to ourselves before his therapy sessions began. I hugged Mylon so tight and told him I'd be back to eat lunch with him. He had tears in his eyes, and it literally broke my heart. While maintaining my emotions, I dug in my purse and gave him a token to keep until I came back. I kissed him, told him to do his best, and not to forget I'd be there with him for lunch. His occupational therapist came and got him so they could start his program for the day. As he was walking off, he kept looking back and waving at me. I didn't move until he turned into his station to start working. Then, I turned to walk out the clinic. Immediately after walking outside, I broke down and cried. I could barely make it to the car before letting out a scream like never before. That cry was long overdue.

At that moment, I submitted completely to God. I thanked God for his unending mercy and grace. I asked Him to keep Mylon covered. I prayed and asked Him to watch over me throughout the day and to watch over Sharee while she was at school. He made a way out of no way, and I'll be forever grateful for that. I cried so hard in my car until I just couldn't cry anymore. Why did this all happen? Why did God choose ME to go through this? All I knew was each day, all I could do was FAITH, Forward All Issues To Him, and keep pressing forward.

Upon arriving at the hotel, I made a list of all the things I needed. There were so many tasks to be accomplished before our trip to North Carolina. Thank God I had this opportunity to get things done. Although my hands were full, I couldn't wait to have lunch with Mylon at noon. I couldn't wait to see him and see how his day was going!

At 11:45 a.m., I was back in the waiting area of the brain injury day treatment clinic. The intake nurse came and got me to get a sneak peek of Mylon. To my surprise, he was participating with a smile. He was moving about the different centers with ease and appeared to be content. When he looked up and saw me, he ran towards me. The smile on his face made me feel at ease; tears ran down my cheeks as I hugged him. I asked him how his day was so far, and he told me it had been great! We had an awesome lunch. He still was having some problems with his gait, so he slobbered quite a bit whenever he ate. Neither of us cared today. It was just so great being able to sit down, eat together and share the feelings of success we both had. It was much easier to say see you later than it was that morning. This time when I told him I would be back to get him at 4:00 p.m., he said, "Ok, mom." He headed down the hall to his stations to begin his afternoon session. Two other kids walked with him, and my heart just filled with joy. I left the hospital with a feeling of ease. Of course, I thanked God for coming through again! The rest of the afternoon was a breeze, and I was able to plan accordingly for my next major move.

When I returned to get Mylon, he was so excited to tell me about his day; I was equally excited to hear it. It was a Friday, so he would not be returning until Monday. The ride to the hotel was great! It was filled with chatter, laughter, excitement and awe! When we got inside, Mylon used the bathroom and climbed onto his bed. He hugged me, told me he loved me and went straight to sleep. My baby had an awesome, yet tiring day. He looked so peaceful as he slept, and I just felt so good at that moment.

I woke him up after two hours so we could go to my sister's house. Since we were leaving the next morning to go to North Carolina, I packed Mylon a bag. It was good to get that out of the way early so I could go straight to sleep after we returned from my sister's. I planned to go get our things Saturday and come straight back to Alabama on Sunday. It would be a long ride, but I was ready for it. We didn't stay at my sister's house long, but we had a great time. Traveling with Mylon was going to be long and tedious, therefore I knew I needed a good night's sleep. We were excited because upon my return, we would be moving into our new apartment. We returned to the hotel and went straight to bed.

The next morning, we woke up and prepared for our trip. To ensure an efficient trip, I made arrangements for someone to travel with us. After getting ready, Mylon and I packed up the car and hit the road. I called my sister before we left so I could talk to my daughter. I told her I loved her and would see her Sunday. We gassed up the car and off to North Carolina we went!

Upon our arrival, it seemed almost unreal. I knew I was on a time line and had no time to waste. So after eating a hearty dinner, we went to the condo and immediately began packing. I sat up an area for Mylon to sleep and due to the long tiring ride, he was asleep in no time. I was happy he was asleep because I needed all the time I could get. Everything from the kitchen utensils to the bed linens were neatly folded and tightly packed away in one of the many boxes I had brought along. After several hours of packing, I realized that it was three in the morning and I needed to get some sleep. So, I laid on the floor next to Mylon and fell fast asleep.

The next morning was a beautiful one. The sunrays shined brightly through the blinds brighter than ever. Being that all the curtains had been packed away was surely a contributing factor. But for some reason, the rays seemed to shine directly in my face. They felt warm, and I almost didn't want to get up. Knowing what was ahead, I had no choice but to get up. I fixed Mylon cereal, got him washed up and dressed so we could start the day.

We left to go get the U-Haul and returned to continue packing. The day went by so fast. And, I must say I was very proud of Mylon. It was almost like he knew I needed him to be on his best behavior and not distract me too much. The entire day, he kept himself entertained by either playing with his toys, watching tv, or taking short cat naps. By 7:00 p.m., it was all done. I taped the last box and put it on the truck. I walked back inside the condo, and it was as empty as it was the day I had moved in it. A bittersweet moment it was. Walking in and out of each room, I couldn't help but think about all that occurred over the past several months. While driving out of the complex, I thanked God yet again for all He had done. We arrived into the hotel and settled in for the night. I was actually looking forward to the next day because to me, it was like the first day of the next chapter for us all.

The alarm clock went off early the next morning. I must have hit the snooze button four or five times. The sun was out again. It was a beautiful morning, and I could hear the birds outside. As I stretched, Mylon sat straight up in the bed, looked at me and said, "It's time to go home." I looked at him and said, "Yes, it is time to go home." We got dressed, grabbed a bite to eat and checked out the hotel. After making sure everything was nice and secure on the U-Haul, we gassed up and prepared to go. As expected, the ride back to Alabama was long and tiring. However, it was a nice, smooth ride. Mylon slept most of the way. Each time I looked in the back seat, he was snuggling his pillow and blanket; his helmet was on and looked as if not to have a care in the world. I loved it!

When I arrived to Alabama, I contacted my sister and told her I was back. My daughter was excited; Mylon and I both couldn't wait to see her. We went straight to our apartment to park the U-Haul for the evening. Afterwards, we went to my sister's, ate dinner and returned back to the apartment for the evening.

Mylon and I were excited to be home. I made a nice pallet on the floor for us to sleep on that night. It was the most comfortable pallet ever. I reminded Mylon that the next day was Monday, which meant he was going back to his program to see his new friends and teachers again. He seemed ok with it, and boy did that make me feel at ease. Well, we settled in for the night and said our prayers. All I could do was think about God's goodness. Through everything, He kept His word to me and didn't leave me for one tiny moment. The moonlight was beautiful. I rolled over, drifted off and slept like a baby. I awakened the next day well rested, rejuvenated and energized. I truly felt like I could tackle the world; and that is exactly what I vowed to do from that day on.

CHAPTER 9

New Beginnings in Another World

Although Mylon experienced his first day of day treatment the previous week, today seemed like it was actually his first day. He was happy and eager to go. I was happy as well because I knew that while he was in the program during the day, I'd be able to get the apartment together. After I dropped him off, I went back home and began to unpack everything. It took me several weeks to unpack everything and get things organized. It didn't matter that things were unorganized at first; it just felt good to be in a place that I could call home. It's an amazing feeling to cook a meal for us, sitting, relaxing, watching TV, and simply taking a long bath in your own space.

I knew it would be an adjustment for my daughter. She had not been around Mylon since he was in ICU. So, things were really new to her. Several thoughts crossed my mind regarding how she would adjust to her baby brother being the way he was now. He wasn't the same Mylon she knew before. I'd often wonder if he had memories of all the fun things they use to do together. Only time would tell. I talked to her about all the things he was doing that he didn't use to do. My goal was to prepare her for what's to come. She needed to understand the severity of his brain injury. It was important to inform her not to take anything personal that he may say or do towards her. It would be challenging, but the one thing we all agreed upon was that no matter what, we'd stick it out together.

Since the apartment had only two bedrooms, Mylon and his sister had to share a room. Initially, I thought them sharing a bedroom wouldn't work out too well, but it actually turned out fine. Mylon normally went to sleep before my daughter, so she normally was able to do any homework or whatever she needed to do without interruptions.

One night, I was in my room and Nasharee was in their room. I had not heard Mylon stirring around, so I walked down the hall into the living room. There he was sitting on the floor doing the unthinkable; Mylon was trying to order an X-rated movie! I yelled his name as loud as I could and said, "NO!!!!" It was all part of the head injury. The doctors warned me about it but my God, I was not expecting to deal with it so soon. Sexual stimulation in head injured persons is usually increased or decreased, and Mylon's seemed to be super increased. From that point on, I had to make sure parental controls were on all televisions and computers. Furthermore, I sat down and explained the rules regarding what to watch and what not to watch on TV.

Weeks passed and things seemed to be getting on track. Routines were being put into play, and Mylon was doing extremely well in the day treatment program. My daughter was doing well in school, made new friends and seemed to be happy. Each night before closing my eyes, I thanked God for all the blessings He had given us and for just being with us each and every day. Life at this moment was good.

Well, most moments were good that is. Mylon began to display some of the actions and behaviors I learned about during his inpatient rehabilitation. Plus, I'd read so many books, articles, and reference guides on traumatic brain injury until I felt that I had a PhD in Traumatic Brain Injury. There were many days filled with agitation, frustrations, violent outburst, and crying spells. Some would refer to it as defiance, but I knew it was all part of the head injury. One day, Mylon jotted out the front door of the apartment, ran down the stairs and across the parking lot into the apartment's rental office. Fear took over me because he didn't have his helmet on, and I didn't want him to fall and hurt himself. That was the day I realized I needed to talk to his doctors about scheduling his next surgery, which was cranial reconstruction. It got to the point where he kept removing his helmet because he didn't want to wear it anymore. During these outbursts, my daughter would often look in awe and not know what to do or say. She tried to be the best big sister she could. She did her best to offer me compassion when she knew I'd had a rough day with Mylon. I loved her dearly for that. My main concern was I didn't want her getting mentally and emotionally drained from all this.

It was indeed more challenging than I ever imagined it would be. Who was this child I had? How could he be so disrespectful and violent towards me? How could he not listen to me when all I ever tried to do was help him? What was going on with my child, and what happened to the quiet Mylon who barely talked when he was in the room? Where was he, and how was I going to raise him to understand that most of the things he was doing was inappropriate? How long would it take for him to get back normal? How long was he going to be this way? How many sleepless nights would I have? How much stress would I be able to endure? How was my daughter going to handle all of this? Who, what, when, where, and how? Those were the questions that bombarded my mind each and every day! “My God, where are you right now?” I wept daily.

It was during this phase of the healing process that I realized all of our lives had indeed been changed forever, and this journey would be everlasting. I prayed and asked God to put all the right people, resources, places and things in position at that time. I didn’t have much to go off of other than knowing that God had not left me. That was enough for me to hold my head up and boldly move forward into our new beginning in another world; a world of the unknown.

CHAPTER 10

God Talks to Me…Do You Believe Me?

The next several months were filled with many miracles. God continued to come through and provide all we needed, just as He promised me He would. The time came for Mylon to have his next major surgery, and he came out great. The morning of his surgery, we got up early because we had to be at the hospital at 6:30 a.m. Once we got ready, I called my mother so they could talk before his surgery. While we were driving, Mylon kept looking up at the sky. At this time of morning, it was pitch black outside, and the sky was filled with stars. It was an oddly clear dawn, and the air was very still. I kept admiring how beautiful the sky was and how the stars seemed to twinkle so bright. Mylon kept looking up, and I finally asked what he was looking at. Calmly turning to me, he said, "I'm looking at the angels. They are touching me." The hairs on my arm stood up and tears began to roll down my face. A feeling of peace came over me like never before. He then looked at me and said, "Do you believe me?" Chills ran through my body as I replied, "Yes." His eyes were filled with tears, and I knew he was sincere.

I smiled at him and couldn't stop looking at him as he smiled back. He looked out the window and quietly said, "God talks to me. He talks to me all the time." I looked at Mylon with a blank stare in my eyes; it was the first time he said anything to me about God since the car accident. What he said to me next was truly a miracle. He said, "When we had the car accident, I died and went to heaven. God told me it wasn't time for me to be there yet, and He was sending me back. But when it was time for me to come, then I would be back." My mouth flew open as tears streamed down my face in sheer awe. I never told him he actually died in my arms in that car wreck, and that he had been revived. He looked at me as I wept and simply asked me again, "Momma, do you believe me?'' I looked at my baby boy, held his hand and answered with a trembling voice, "Yes, I most certainly do." At that moment life stood still, and without a doubt, I then knew that on June 18, 2001, God was surely right there with us in the car after the accident.

Regarding his surgery and hospital stay, well I think you know the outcome. It was an awesome recovery, and his cranial reconstruction went well. The surgery enabled him to wear his baseball caps and not that dreadful helmet. When we left the hospital, the huge indention and soft spot was no longer on his head!! They took a piece of his skull from the opposite side and split it like an oreo cookie. From there, they reconstructed it to fit the side where his skull was removed after the accident. He looked great. We were both happy. It took a while for all the swelling to go down and for his hair to grow back. Once it did grow back, oh boy, he was one happy camper.

Several more months passed, and it was time for his day treatment program to come to an end. The many days of physical therapy, occupational therapy, speech, and more finally paid off. He was able to use his right side much better than he had before. And, his speech…my God he was talking too much now! Although there was still an impediment, it was awesome that he was capable of communicating with me and say what he wanted to say with less trouble. The exit interview for the program went well. Mylon excelled in every area he was evaluated in; his progress was phenomenal!

Since Mylon did so well, they had surprising news in store for him. "You hear that you're going back to school?" they asked. He looked at me and gave me the biggest smile ever. While saying our goodbyes, Mylon gave out hugs like it was candy; I simply couldn't thank them enough for saving my son. Walking out of that hospital was a huge sigh of relief. Coming to Alabama for his outpatient care was the best decision I made.

CHAPTER 11

The Transformation

What was school going to be like for this little boy? This was among the many thoughts racing through my mind while we drove home. Regardless of my fears, it was a step we needed to take.

The next week, I contacted the school and explained our situation. They arranged a time for me to bring Mylon to the school and speak with the guidance counselor in regards to enrollment.

At the time of the accident, he just completed the sixth grade and was going to the seventh grade. They enrolled him into the seventh grade, but my gut kept telling me to start him back over in the sixth. To this day, I wish I would've listened to my intuition regarding that decision. It was agreed upon he would go to school half-days and be in the resource room. He was still required to wear his helmet for a few hours a day but was allowed to wear a baseball cap for the rest of the day. Although he was well aware of the fact he had to wear the helmet, he really had no insight as to why. Kids teased him, which made him hate school. On top of that, he was placed in the special education resource room for his classes. Prior to the accident, he was an honor roll student who made all A's and B's. He remembered this and often refused to go into the classroom. This became the norm as far as school was concerned.

The kids in the resource room were very nice to him, but he just didn't seem to fit in. Luckily, he eventually enjoyed being around the other kids. Even though he didn't fully understand why he was in the resource room, he knew it was a place different from what he was used to in school.

The first several weeks were tedious for him. Those half-days were tiresome for him. It never failed; as soon as I picked him up at noon each day, he'd get in the car and fall fast asleep. He developed a unique taste for chicken. The routine was to get him chicken so he would have to eat when he woke up. It was like clockwork and became our routine for several months. He didn't really learn much during those half-days, but the socialization did him a world of good. Just being able to be around other kids was truly enough for him. I admit it was enough for me, too.

As the end of the year approached, I got a phone call from my chain of command. They informed me about my assignment to the closest Army installation, which happened to be in

Huntsville, Alabama. So, that meant I'd have to go back to North Carolina to clear my unit. I spent the next few weeks preparing to go back to sign out of my unit and sign into the new one. I informed Mylon's teacher that he'd be out a couple of days.

We drove back to Fayetteville, North Carolina on a Monday morning. This time, the ride didn't seem as long. Maybe because Mylon was able to take in the scenery, as well as adjust himself and maneuver around in the back seat on his own. It made such a big difference.

After making it to North Carolina safe and sound, we checked into our hotel. I contacted my supervisor to inform him I was there and got my instructions for the next few days. At this time, not an ounce or worry consumed me; I actually felt quite grateful. What the Army did for me was truly unheard of. They allowed me to go off for almost a year and care for my son without any hassles whatsoever. Who does that?

The next morning, Mylon and I got prepared for the long day. When I arrived to my unit, everyone seemed so happy to see me. And, I was equally happy to see them. I thanked them from the depths of my soul for all the support and prayers they gave my family and I.

Clearing the unit was a breeze. It only took me two days, because they had already taken care of almost everything for me. I will never forget Command Sergeant Major (CSM) Norris Hand and my Dragon Brigade Family. Without them, there is no way I would have been able to make it. I truly thank God for them all. As I drove off the installation, there was one last thing I just had to do. I had to go by Cape Fear Hospital to see the staff who worked so diligently on Mylon while he was there.

I drove down Reily Road, the street where the accident occurred. Flashbacks began to return. My mind replayed everything that happened that day... step-by-step, play-by-play. It felt gut wrenching, but I had to do it. I trembled as I drove past the spot where we once were covered in glass and blood. The hairs on my arm stood up, and I could hear the crash and the sirens. I could see all the people standing around. I was actually reliving that moment all over again. On the other hand, Mylon didn't have a clue where we were, nor did he realize what was taking place within me. And, I was glad he didn't.

When we arrived at Cape Fear Hospital, so many memories bombarded me. I parked, then Mylon and I walked in. I explained to him that this was where he was after the accident, and he didn't remember one single thing. We went upstairs to the PICU so he could see the bare floor I slept on before they gave me a room. I then took him to the inpatient rehabilitation area. To our surprise, some of the nurses, doctors and speech therapist who worked with Mylon were on shift. One of the nurses saw us; she ran toward us and hugged Mylon as she wept uncontrollably. The speech therapist looked at me with tears running down her face and said, "This can't be the same person who was here in this hospital with me." They all could not believe how far Mylon had come and how well he looked.

By the time the doctor came over to us, we all were in tears while hugging each other. He shook Mylon's hand and asked him if he knew who he was. Of course, Mylon shook his head no. From there, I explained who everyone was. He really didn't know what to say to anyone but then again, he really didn't need to. It was a very emotional moment for us all, and one that I will never forget. After about an hour, we said our goodbyes and departed the hospital. Not a dry eye was in the group that waved as we drove off, including mines and Mylon's. We didn't say much on the way to gas up. In my heart, I somehow knew something pretty amazing had taken place.

We made it back to Alabama safely and began to prepare for the next part of our journey.

CHAPTER 12

An Everlasting Smile

Over the next few years, Mylon grew stronger and stronger. However, we did face many more challenges. School was a major challenge but with hard work and perseverance, he made it through. I vowed to never let anyone tell him that he was incapable of doing what others could do; he could be whatever he wanted in life. I taught him that life wasn't going to be easy for him, but with God all things would be possible.

He made it through middle school. Due to me being in the military, we moved quite a bit. Fortunately, he met many people along the way. Some good, some not so good, but each one brought about a learning experience. High school was a huge challenge. Plenty of time was spent with IEP's and fighting to make sure the school system didn't stick him in special education classrooms. Although it was a draining process, it had to be done. Most of his teachers were true to heart and really cared about making a difference. On the other hand, there were some who made statements to me such as, "Why can't he be put in special education classrooms with other people like him?" Or, "He's going to fail my class because he's not going to be able to keep up." I truly thank them the most, especially his eighth-grade teacher who gave me one of my most challenging task as his caregiver. Their actions motivated me to never give up, which in turn allowed me to teach Mylon the same.

Watching him play on the school's basketball team and making only one point the entire season was priceless. Watching him having to wear a baseball cap every single day to school was sometimes hard because kids would tease him or ask him why he had to wear them. Unfortunately, he could never attend school functions, such as basketball games, football games, track meets, school dances, or his senior prom. It was all too stimulating for him. Due to his lack of socialization skills, it was difficult for him to not become frustrated or agitated. Sitting through IEP meetings and listening to school administrators tell me we should settle for him getting a high school certificate instead of striving to get a regular diploma was frustrating. It showed they didn't really believe in his potential, but it didn't matter because I did.

Guess what? Mylon graduated with a regular diploma a semester early. He was unable to walk with his class because the military relocated us to South Carolina before the graduation ceremony.

Not taking him back to participate in his graduation is another decision I will always regret. However, his diploma proudly sits on his bedroom dresser. Many days, I stare at it and thank God for giving us both the drive to keep going. Even though he doesn't know what it took for him to achieve it, it's a constant reminder to me of how our hard work paid off.

One thing he did take away from his high school years was the nickname Smiley. Mylon was one who always smiled. It was his smile that everyone referred to him by. No matter what kind of day he was having, he'd smile. He could be frustrated, in pain, or having the worst day ever, but it didn't matter. His smile would never escape his face. All the teachers, friends, doctors and acquaintances he met saw his smile before they saw anything else. To this day, it's still a huge part of who he is. It's warm, inviting and melts your heart. For me, it's a constant reminder that God is always there with us…but especially him. To this day, it's still what people say attracts them to him. You see it's through his smile that he's able to show you the miracle that he truly is. It's through his smile he shows you all that God has done for him. It's through his smile that he is reminded God will remain by his side. It's through his smile that I find strength to keep pushing, even on days when no one knows how bad I want to give up and quit. My Smiley and his everlasting smile is truly what keeps me from not giving up this caregiver's fight. It somehow seems to always brighten my darkest days. Trust me, I still have many.

CHAPTER 13

X's and O's

2007 was a year that love was definitely in the air. For me, having dealt with all that had transpired alone had really taken a toll on me. In 2005 after my divorce, someone I'd dated years ago found out about our accident and reached out to me. I felt he resurfaced at a time when I was in a very low place. His genuine care and concern drew me as it was what I had been missing for quite some time. Our conversations and time together became refreshing and it was as if we never had any time apart.

You see, I had forgotten about me! My life had been put on hold since our accident. The devastation that I was enduring was already enough but having to divorce an abusive spouse through the midst of it all was just too much for one person to bear. However, God kept me sane and brought me through.

With Dexter, life became better because I felt that now I didn't have to fight this fight alone. Actually having someone to lean on and not always being the strong tower of strength for others to lean on was a great feeling. Years passed and it became more apparent that he was there for a reason, and that reason was to be there just for me. We married on February 16, 2007. As for Mylon, relationships in high school were something that he really was unable to handle. The socialization skills he lacked always interfered with him being able to maintain normal healthy friendships. Most days, simply going to school and making it through the day was a difficult task. With that being said, he never got to experience what it felt like to have a high school sweetheart. Well, not until we moved to South Carolina anyway.

The move from where he attended high school was a huge transition for him. Having to adjust to making new friends and meeting new people was always a task for Mylon. He never met a stranger beforehand. However, because he did not "look" like he had a head injury; people normally could not understand his actions and would shy away from him. He was often left spending days, nights, and weekends alone without any friends.

South Carolina was where Mylon met his first true love. She came from a very loving family, who all loved Mylon and treated him great. It was like she was God-sent, if you will. She displayed the patience needed to deal with Mylon. She never got frustrated or agitated with him. Constantly, I'd wonder, "Where did this girl come from?"

Their relationship was so cute. Her mother would bring her to our house often to see Mylon, and they would watch tv in the living room for hours. Sometimes, she would even cook him his favorite meal...fried chicken. My husband and I thanked God for her because what she was able to bring into our son's life was priceless. He was able to attend functions with her; state fairs, and even was able to conduct himself like a gentleman when they went to dinner or the movies, most times anyway. Life was grand because my son was experiencing a part of life that he wanted so badly; to have a young lady in his life who accepted him for him, brain injury and all. Her selflessness was phenomenal.

She was a senior in high school and a star student. As her school year came to an end, it was time for her senior prom. I will never forget the conversation she and I had regarding her prom. Since he was not able to attend his senior prom and experience the joys it brought to his other classmates, she wanted her prom to be about HIM I will never forget the feeling I had when she told me that. She was every mother's dream; an unselfish, dependable, reliable, trustworthy, and most of all loving young lady. What mom would not want her to be in their son's life?

The weeks planning for the prom were awesome and exciting for them both. Seeing the excitement on Mylon's face each day as they planned their color scheme for the prom and other festivities were invaluable. The joy he experienced was like no other.

Prom day finally arrived, and they were the most beautiful couple there. The brown and beige they choose was breathtakingly beautiful, and she looked like a true princess in her gown. Mylon looked so debonair in his suit. As he watched out of the front door waiting for her to get there, tears ran down my face. At that moment, I saw my baby boy as a young man for the first time since our accident. Their evening had some challenges. Being the superstar his girlfriend was, she did not waiver. The sacrifices she made that evening allowed Mylon to enjoy himself, as if he was the only person in the world who mattered that night.

They continued to see each other throughout the summer. We took trips to the beach and spent tons of family time together. As the summer came to an end, it was time for her to leave for college. She was accepted into a college that was about three hours away. This was difficult for them both, but we understood her future could not be put on hold.

She and Mylon tried really hard to continue their relationship. He was unable to comprehend the fact that she went away to school; he became frustrated and agitated because of it. It became too much for them to deal with, so they ended their relationship. This was a very difficult time for Mylon. He became quiet and withdrawn. It took some time but things started to get back to normal. As time passed on, so did his solemnity. Soon, his signature smile returned. He eventually began to get involved with some of the local brain injury support groups and his life started over.

The Brain Injury Association of South Carolina provided some of the best social rehabilitation Mylon ever received. Their support group was full of educational sessions for the survivor as well as the caregiver. It was the first time Mylon opened up and spoke openly about our car accident. It provided a fun environment, and was comprised of survivors within his age range. For the first time he felt comfortable and not like an outsider. It came at a time when he truly needed it most.

"How do I love thee? Let me count the ways." There were just too many, and we will always love this young lady. Every time we reminisce about her, Mylon still smiles. That lets me know she and her family will always hold a special place in his heart and mine.

CHAPTER 14

Sky's the Limit...Let the Marathon Begin

He began therapy which turned out to be much more rewarding than we ever imagined. During his daily sessions, he built an awesome relationship with his occupational therapist. Mylon would come home and enthusiastically tell me how easy it was to talk to him. As time passed, I just had to meet who he referred to as his super therapist.

One day, I went to pick up Mylon and arrived early to inconspicuously observe him. What I saw was simply amazing. I saw Mylon not only working hard on his own, but he was also helping others. His OT would give him instructions, and he would follow through with ease. There was a passion in Mylon's eyes that I had not seen in a very long time. So after his session, I introduced myself to his OT and thanked him for being the super therapist that we so often called him. He told me his name was Dan and how they all loved working with Mylon. It was apparent, Mylon had won their hearts. His drive to work hard and persevere impressed everyone. His willingness to assist the other patients upon completion of his therapy sessions was so important to him. Dan and the others assured me that his success there would be inevitable. At that moment, God showed me that Mylon was definitely in good hands with Dan.

Months and months passed, and Mylon continued to do well during his day treatment program. His OT came to me and inquired if I thought Mylon would do some volunteer work at the facility. I thought it was an awesome idea! It would not only give him some working skills, but it would also assist him with some of the social skills he still tremendously lacked. With Dan there to mentor him, I knew it would be a great thing for Mylon to do. Fortunately, Mylon ended up getting approved. His responsibility consisted of transporting patients from their rooms down to the gym for their therapy sessions. Each day, he would perform his job with a smile on his face; he truly enjoyed every moment. The patients and staff all loved him because he brought a sense of peace and joy to all he met. Dan and his family became a permanent fixture in Mylon's and my life. Much of his time was spent with the Carroll family playing basketball, helping coach, and even going to church with them. Their birthdays are even on the same day! Dan became one of the many blessings that God had sent our way. To this day, we both have his number on speed dial and communicate with him often.

As I fast forward, years have passed and life itself has become more and more difficult. Well, I guess it would be fair to say we've had some good days and we've had some hills to climb; but through it all, we won't complain.

Mylon experienced his first seizure in 2003 while we were in the car. While having a conversation, he began to stutter; well at least that's what I thought he was doing. It puzzled me because I never saw him do it before.

It occurred once again the following week, so I contacted his doctor. After sending us to a neurologist and conducting tests, we learned he was experiencing interrupted complex partial seizures. "Seizures…oh no!" I thought to myself. The seizures continued but were controlled by medication.

It wasn't until 2007 that he had his first Grand mal seizure. It scared me out of my mind! I walked into his room, and he was slumped over the bed with half of his body on the floor. He wasn't responsive, and I screamed for my husband to come upstairs and call 911. After calling, my husband carried him downstairs while we waited on the ambulance. He slowly regained awareness, but it was one of the scariest moments I'd ever experienced.

In addition to the seizures, his behavior changed drastically. The once quiet as a mouse son I had was now loud and impulsive. He still had some major problems with aphasia. This language disorder was caused by the injury to his left frontal lobe. The left side of the brain is dominant for language in most people. Therefore if injured, it can cause major problems with speaking, listening, reading, and writing. Mylon's aggressiveness and impulsiveness grew from week to week. It was extremely hard seeing my baby this way. My heart wouldn't allow me to yell at him or be angry when he did things he wasn't supposed to do. I tried my best to keep in mind it was the head injury contributing to most of his mishaps. He got into several altercations until one day; I just couldn't take the stress anymore.

I contacted his doctor and asked if she thought medication management would be beneficial. She suggested several options and to much avail, it was just what he needed. Now don't get me wrong, Mylon still experiences days of frustration, impulsion and aggression. But, I have learned to cope with these times by diverting his attention when these incidents occur. You must understand that after the initial injury, many traumatic brain injury symptoms aren't visible to a stranger's glance. Most people are used to seeing casts on broken bones, missing limbs on amputees, or bandages on burn victims. But, traumatic brain injury symptoms are normally only visible to close family members. Some signs for me are seeing him forget what he was saying or finding difficulty in expressing himself. There are many times when I catch Mylon looking at me during an event or when he's speaking to someone. I know what each glance in my direction means. A drooping shoulder while someone is talking signifies he's struggling to find the right words; while a gleam in his eyes indicates he had a complete conversation without any difficulties.

It is now 2017, and so much has happened. Some things good, and some things not so good. In 2016 he experienced a few seizures which were definitely setbacks. While tears rolled down my face, all I could do was think to myself, "God, not again."

Through it all, this has been one heck of a journey. Mylon has experienced love, heartbreak, college, jobs...you name it, and he's pretty much experienced it. Life has been hard for him. Finding friends has been one of the toughest things he has gone through.

He took his first college class in 2007. We were living in South Carolina, and he wanted so badly to attend college. So, I enrolled him into the local technical college there. It was a struggle for him to stay on task; his inability to actually comprehend the level of work made it difficult for him to stay engaged and interested in the classwork. This brought about other frustrations, which led to the breakdown in his socialization skills. Eventually, he had to be withdrawn from the school. Socialization was and still is difficult, however we've found mechanisms to cope.

He is currently enrolled at the local technical college. Each time he comes to me and says he wants to take a class, we encourage him to simply do the best he can.

There's still difficulty in making friends, not knowing what to say and when to say it. Even after 15 years, he still has restless nights. Through it all, we are still learning new things every day. Each day we experience various victories and defeats. We have learned to take the good with the bad and keep striving.

His ability to get jobs has been good; his inability to maintain the job causes him grief. Several services have been put in place to assist. We are always hopeful that one day, he will obtain gainful employment. In Mylon's words, he will maintain a "grown man's job".

His dating life has been...well, let's just say quite a roller coaster. He's met some pretty interesting young ladies. Some have great intentions, while others don't. His big heart normally prevents him from spotting the ones who really don't have his best interest in mind. There are some who make "mama bear" surface, which they all end up not liking. He has experienced some horror stories, as well as some awesome love stories.

He's obtained some awesome mentors who have invested hours of time and prayers into his journey. Failures have been experienced but through it all, he has been able to push through with a determination like no other. He has touched the lives of others, whether it's with his loving personality or beautiful smile that brightens the darkest room. His resilience has helped me and others tremendously. Mylon is living proof that with God, all things are indeed possible. He has a love for music and will sing no matter who's around. His heart to please and serve is another characteristic I love; he will do almost anything to help others in need.

Several times a day, he comes to me and expresses his dreams and goals. Like any other 28-year-old, he expresses his desires to live on his own and have a family. I've watched him cry, laugh, and fight to the end. Despite the obstacles he faces on a daily basis, he wakes up every morning like it's his very first day on Earth. We have learned what works and what doesn't work. Things like following strict routines can be the difference in a great day versus a day filled with frustrations. Teaching him that sleep has to be a priority has been quite a challenge, but setting specific times for certain activities has been beneficial. Knowing what time to take medicine, eat, or have quiet time establishes the structure he needs in his life. Life after brain injury is one full of ups and downs.

In regards to God, I know God does indeed talk to him. The promise God made to me regarding healing Mylon was true. I know his future is bright. Without a doubt, God is with him. No matter what may come, he will not give up and will stay the course. I know the little boy who God saved back in 2001 is now a man after God's own heart. Because he truly loves God, no weapon that forms against him will prosper. He will be successful at whatever God brings his way.

As I write these pages, I think of each and every person whose life is affected by brain injury.

Many families face the same gloom and dark days as we do. From experience, I know it brings life-threatening hardships, burdens, anguish and distress. I pray that HOPE still lives in their hearts. It is hope for better days ahead that keeps our faith and spirit alive and our souls in motion.

Yes, the doctors were right about one thing; my son is not the same person he was before the accident. But hey, neither am I. I prefer to interact with as few people as possible. I am jumpy and extra watchful whenever I'm in a car. Often, I think about life and try to make sense of death, pain, suffering, and most of all heartache. Even though I don't ask as much as I did before, I still wonder why God let this happen to Mylon and not me. Even through all my anger and pain, I know God is noticeably here with us. No matter the circumstance, He never fails me. In his power, might and even His simplicity, He's always there.

I find myself yearning for His voice through the splendor of the heavens. The skies literally talk with its sunsets, sunrises and arrays of breathtaking colors such as orange, yellow, purple and gold. I listen for His whispers through the movement of the trees with each wind that blows. He converses in the shape of the clouds as they waltz across the sky before dissolving. Raindrops and thunder speak like no other. I look for God's voice in my grandkids' laughter and the I love you's escaping my children's mouths. I look for Him in others when I look into their eyes or see them smiling. I look for Him through the kindness of others or my husband's hugs and kisses. I look for Him in the oceans as I watch the waves come in one after the other. In other words, I look for Him everywhere. Although He has not given me any answers as to why this happened, I always feel His presence and comfort when I need it the most.

It has been 15 years since our car accident, and I am still unable to fully verbalize my grief, sorrow and pain. I could write for days, months, and even years and still not truly capture what my heart feels. Nonetheless, when I see my son's smile each day, it reminds me that God's amazing grace is everywhere. It reminds me of the conversation he had with God when He told him it wasn't time for him to come to heaven yet. As I finish this book, we will continue waiting to see what normal is going to be for Mylon. Remember, he wants to live independently, and I want him to. Knowing that time is in God's hands, I know He will grant Mylon the desires of his heart and mold him into what He wants him to be.

He still struggles with the seizures, lack of socialization skills, and other things that TBI survivors struggle with. Often, he says his head injury ruined his life; I simply remind him that his life is merely changed and not ended. He still has the smile that landed him the nickname of Smiley. Every day, he wakes up and chooses to have the best life he can. Yes, life is still full of frustration, anger, pain and disappointments. However, when I see the smile on his face, I hug him and remind him that I love him with all of my heart. As his mother, caregiver, best friend and his biggest advocate, I encourage him not to give up.

To everyone reading this, especially caregivers, hang in there and know with God all things are possible. At times, it's difficult for me to see the struggles he goes through and the tears he sheds. Or to hear him talk about not wanting to live because he's so overwhelmed with frustration because of the way he views himself or is misunderstood by others. No mother wants to see her child go through tough times. Regardless, Mylon always has a sense of resiliency; he can overcome any obstacle that approaches him. His smile is a constant reminder that God answered my prayer on June 18, 2001…the day our lives were changed forever.

Mylon,

I want you to know that you can do all things through Christ who gives you the strength to get up each day and keep going. The best is yet to come son! I will always love you and be here to encourage you every step of the way.

Scriptures That Kept Me Strong and Brought Me Through

Isaiah 53:5 KJV "But He was wounded for our transgressions, He was bruised for our iniquities; The chastisement for our peace was upon Him, And by His stripes we are healed."

Matthew 11:28 KJV "Come unto me all who are weary and burdened, and I will give you rest."

Matthew 14:14 KJV "I am moved with compassion toward the sick and I heal them."

Mark 9:23 KJV "If you can believe, all things are possible to him that believeth".

I Peter 2:24 KJV "By MY stripes you were healed."

Psalms 147:3 KJV "He heals the brokenhearted, and binds up their wounds."

James 5:14, 15 KJV "Is anyone among you sick? Let him call for the elders of the church, and let them pray over him, anointing him with oil in the name of the Lord. And the prayer of faith will save the sick, and the Lord will raise him up. And if he has committed sins, he will be forgiven."

Psalms 91:14-16 KJV "Because he loves me," says the LORD, "I will rescue him; I will protect him, for he acknowledges my name. He will call upon me, and I will answer him; I will be with him in trouble, I will deliver him and honor him. With long life will I satisfy him and show him my salvation."

Matthew 18:18-20 KJV "I tell you the truth, whatever you bind on earth will be bound in heaven, and whatever you loose on earth will be loosed in heaven. Again, I tell you that if two of you on earth agree about anything you ask for, it will be done for you by my Father in heaven. For where two or three come together in my name, there am I with them."

Mark 11:24 KJV "Therefore I tell you, whatever you ask for in prayer, believe that you have received it, and it will be yours."

John 14:14 KJV "If ye shall ask anything in my name, I will do it."

Revelation 12:11 KJV "They overcame him by the blood of the Lamb and by the word of their testimony."

2 Kings 20:5 KJV "I have heard your prayer and seen your tears; I will heal you."

Hosea 6:1-3 KJV "Come, and let us return unto the LORD: for he hath torn, and he will heal us; he hath smitten, and he will bind us up. After two days will he revive us: in the third day he will raise us up, and we shall live in his sight. Then shall we know, if we follow on to know the LORD: his going forth is prepared as the morning; and he shall come unto us as the rain, as the latter and the former rain unto the earth.

Images of Broken Wings

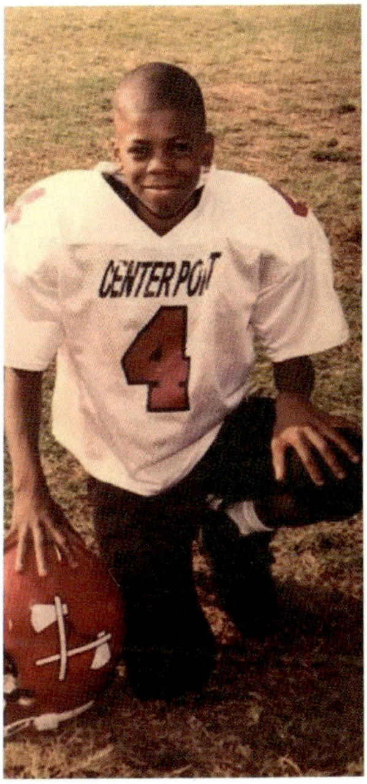

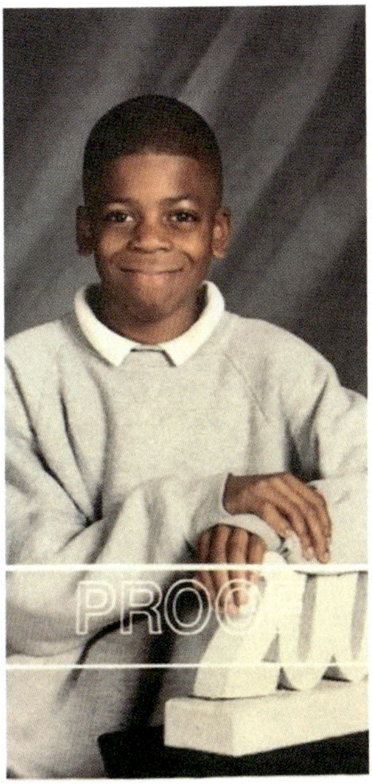

Mylon at ages 10 & 11

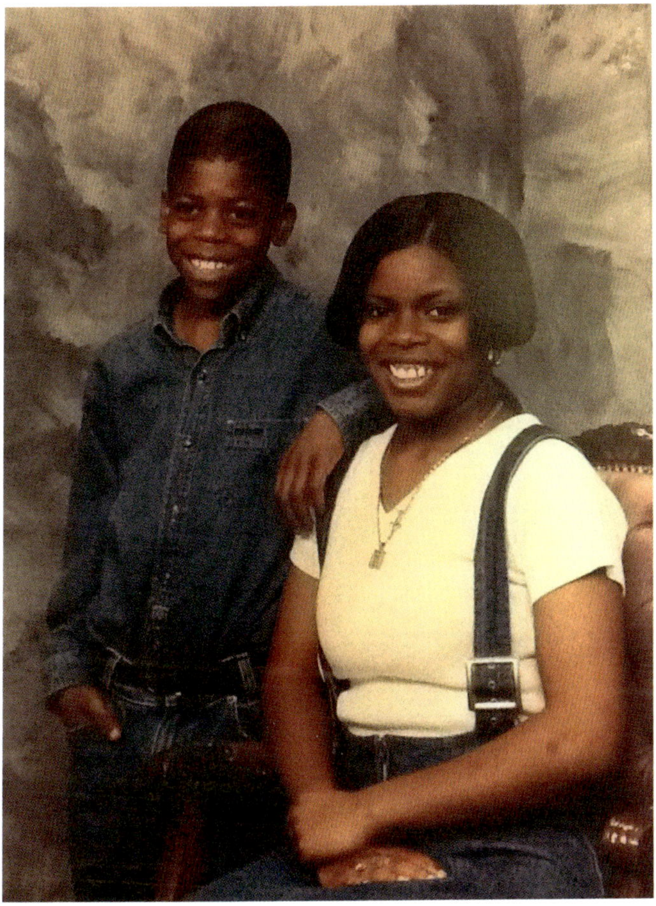

Mylon & Nasharee

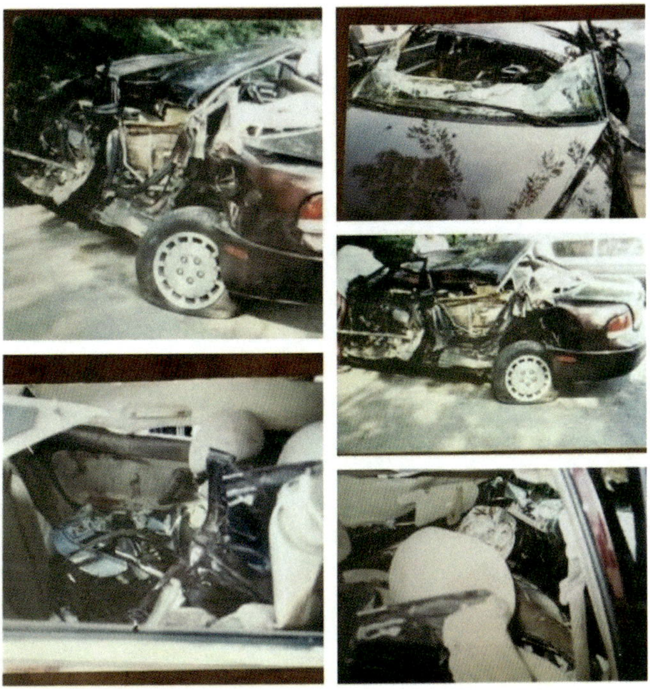

The day our lives changed forever

June 18, 2001

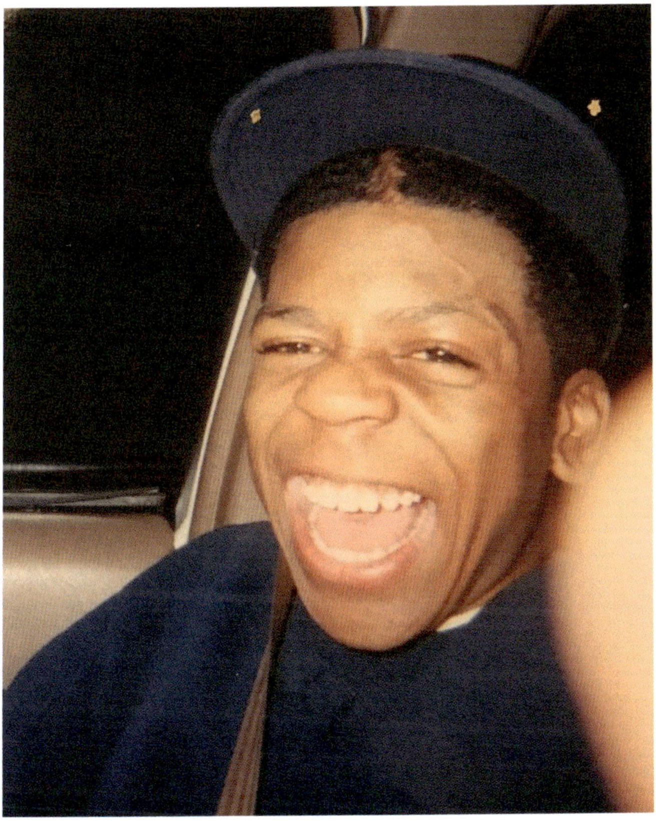

Smiley

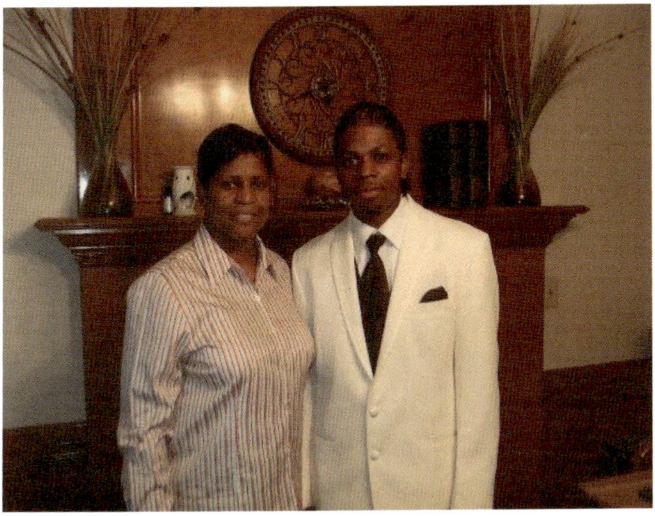

Prom Time (proud Mom)

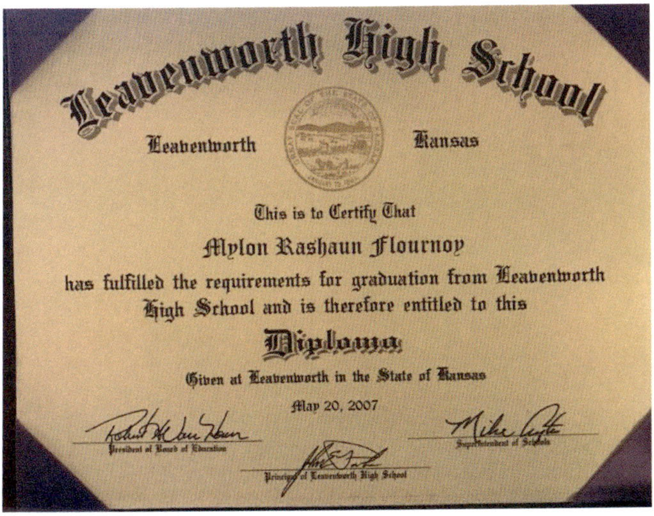

Leavenworth High School

Leavenworth Kansas

This is to Certify That

Mylon Rashaun Flournoy

has fulfilled the requirements for graduation from Leavenworth High School and is therefore entitled to this

Diploma

Given at Leavenworth in the State of Kansas

May 20, 2007

President of Board of Education

Superintendent of Schools

Principal of Leavenworth High School

Mylon's Diploma

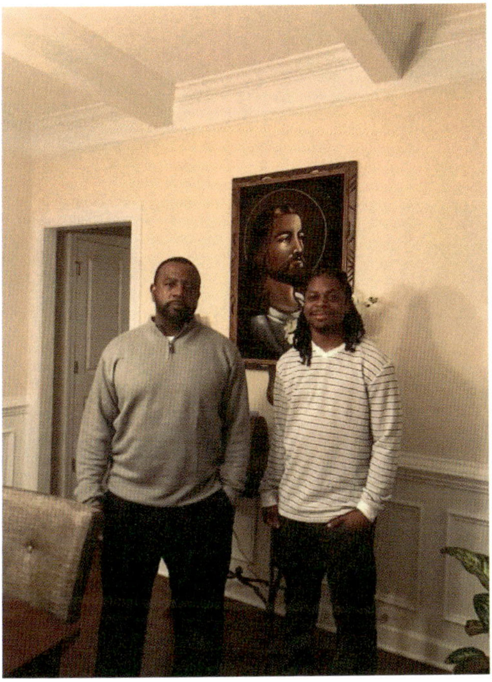

Mylon & Dad

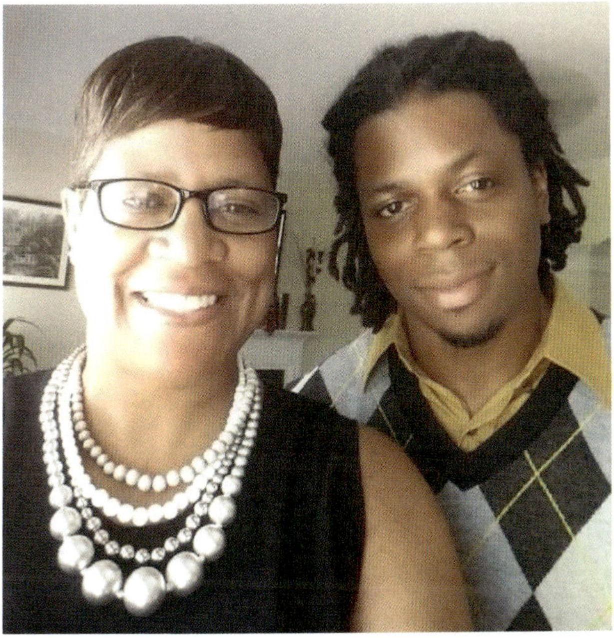

Mylon & Mom

His Caregiver & Biggest Fan

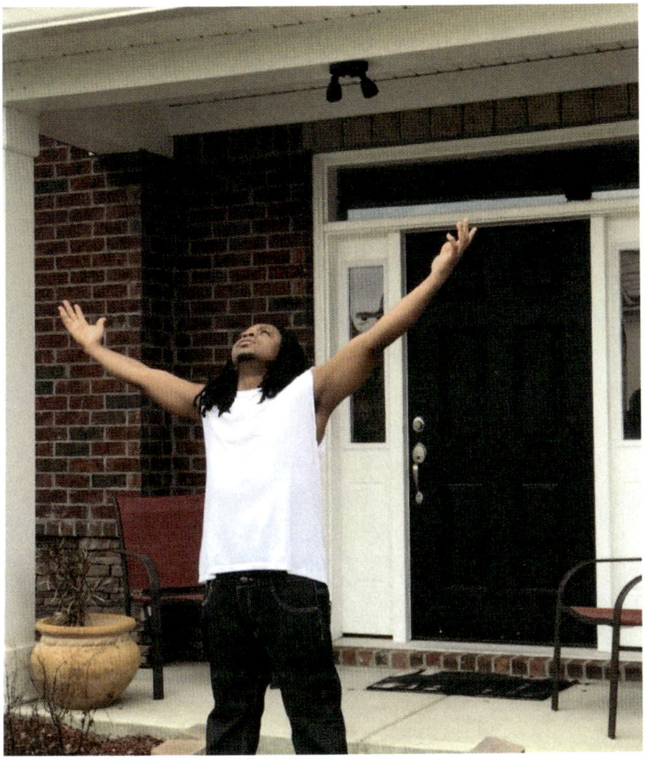

About the Author

Born in Columbus, Mississippi Twylia Reid lives in Savannah, Ga, with her husband Dexter and son Mylon. They're a blended family of 4 adult children and 5 grandchildren. She is a graduate of Trident University International with a bachelor of science in Business Management. She is a US Army retiree of 20 years, a minister, business owner, conference speaker and devoted brain injury advocate.

For book signing and speaking requests:

Websites: www.twyliareid.com/
& www.whenheavenspeaks.net
Email: brokenwings0618@gmail.com
Facebook: www.facebook.com/authortwyliareid/
Linked In: www.linkedin.com/in/twyliareid